A Doctor's Path

A Doctor's Path

◆

Lessons I've Learned on My Journey through Practicing Medicine

Ernie Pellegrino Jr., MD

iUniverse, Inc.

New York Bloomington Shanghai

A Doctor's Path
Lessons I've Learned on My Journey through Practicing Medicine

iUniverse books may be ordered through booksellers or by contacting:

iUniverse
1663 Liberty Drive
Bloomington, IN 47403
www.iuniverse.com
1-800-Authors (1-800-288-4677)

Because of the dynamic nature of the Internet, any Web addresses or links contained in this book may have changed since publication and may no longer be valid.

The information, ideas, and suggestions in this book are not intended as a substitute for professional medical advice. Before following any suggestions contained in this book, you should consult your personal physician. Neither the author nor the publisher shall be liable or responsible for any loss or damage allegedly arising as a consequence of your use or application of any information or suggestions in this book.

ISBN: 978-0-595-47934-4 (pbk)
ISBN: 978-0-595-71966-2 (cloth)

Printed in the United States of America

For my wife, Barbara, whose sacrifices during our entire marriage have made my medical career and family life possible and fulfilling.

Contents

Preface

Doctors often have one thing in common. They tend to have strong opinions about the practice of medicine and the individuals they have met through their vocation. I am no exception. What I have tried to do here is without question judgmental. Some may question my qualifications. I feel my education and training at a leading Midwestern university and medical school, as well as attaining the position of associate clinical professor of orthopedic surgery, responsible for evaluating and training the University of Wisconsin residents in orthopedic surgery, lend credence to those qualifications. I have also had the responsibility of being the chair of the orthopedic department of a two-hundred-plus multispecialty group. My experience on the credentials committee of St. Mary's Hospital in Madison, WI, required me to evaluate numerous physicians. Later I was the chair of the Department of Surgery and chief of staff of St. Mary's Hospital, which has won numerous awards for quality of care. Finally, being a member of the Midwest Regional Committee of the American Academy of Orthopedic Surgery, which evaluated applicants to the Academy, gave me particular insight into the qualifications required of candidates.

Everyone makes mistakes; no one is perfect. As individuals, we all need to be alert for potential mistakes, but it becomes even more important to be aware when someone is trying to cover up or ignore those mistakes. When doctors make mistakes, it can result in damage to the ones placed in our trust. It is critical that we have in place a means of identifying, correcting, and preventing mistakes from happening again. I think medicine has come a long way since I graduated from medical school in 1964, but, unless we are constantly proactive in this regard, we may fail to protect those we have pledged to help.

It is not my purpose to offend. Neither am I writing this to become popular with all of the medical profession. I am far enough removed now, with the exception of the free clinic for the uninsured that I started over five years ago, to feel any pain from writing this. My hope is that, through reading my story, young doctors, medical students, and individuals thinking about medicine as a profession will learn something. Chances are I will not likely influence many long-standing professionals (doctors) by what I have written. Many in the latter group have likely taken a similar journey of their own.

Lastly, it is my intention to show that in medicine, as in all professions, there is a spectrum of individuals who vary from noble to seriously flawed. Additionally, I hope to give my readers some ideas on what to look for and ask of their doctors to obtain the best possible treatment for their medical and psychological problems.

About the Author

After twenty-nine years of active medical practice and eight years of volunteer medical work in Africa and in the United States, I have reflected on my experiences as a board-certified orthopedic surgeon in a high-caliber Midwestern medical community and my practice in the Air Force. The journey you will take through this book is one that I have taken myself. What you see will be in large part colored by my heritage, upbringing, and training. I hope you come away with the notion that men and women who are noble and humble, but not without their flaws, serve the practice of medicine. I have taken the liberty of changing the names of some of the individuals in this book to prevent embarrassment and to avoid any nuisance litigation, despite the fact that everything I have written is true to the best of my knowledge. I have noted where these name changes take place by surrounding the fictitious name in quotation marks.

To understand where I am coming from, it is important to understand something of my personal background. I am the oldest of six children in a working-class Italian family. During my childhood, my worst act of mischief was stealing ripe cherries at night from a neighborhood fruit tree planted close to one of the alleys that ran through each block in the area. My father worked in an assembly line for the Simmons mattress factory in Kenosha, WI. My mother was a seamstress for the Jockey Company. In addition to the family tradition of hard work, we were all well rooted in the local Roman Catholic church, which served primarily an Italian, German, and Polish immigrant population.

Excelling in academics, music, and athletics made it possible for me to get partial college scholarships from the local Elks Club and neighboring Johnson Wax Foundation in Racine, WI. My savings from numerous odd jobs supplemented these scholarships. I delivered newspapers, shined shoes in a shoe parlor, sold ice cream bars from a tricycle ice cream delivery box that I rode all over town, set bowling pins, worked in a foundry, mowed roadside grass and patched blacktop pot holes for the county highway department, and played trumpet for dances in a small instrumental combo that included my very talented younger brother, Ron. The only way Dad could afford to pay for our eight to ten years of lessons was by working a second job as a bartender for a busy bowling alley/restaurant.

I decided to go to college without any hesitation, but deciding on the purpose of my college education was not so simple. Some of my high school teachers wanted me to go into academics, particularly my English teacher, for whom I had done some creative writing that she liked. My decision, however, was made indirectly by my mother's illness. She had been suffering from the effects of breast cancer and its treatment during my entire junior year and until January of my senior year in high school, when she died. This left a horrible gap in our large family, and my youngest sibling was only four. This heart-wrenching experience pushed me to become a doctor and work on developing a cure for cancer. I wanted no one else to see his or her mother or loved one suffer and waste away as we had with our mother. This purpose carried me through my college and early medical school years. I drove myself to succeed—no matter how difficult it might be.

My father did not have the resources to send me or my brothers and sisters to college, but he continued to pledge a weekly allowance of five dollars to use as we wished. In addition to the small scholarships and my savings from the jobs previously described, I supplemented this money during my undergraduate years with odd jobs on campus, such as maintaining vending machines and tending bar for dormitory weekend beer parties. My many jobs gave me a great appreciation of the value of the dollar.

I started my undergraduate work at the University of Wisconsin in Madison in the fall of 1957. At that time I was most appreciative of the accelerated program the medical school made available that allowed a student to become eligible to enter medical school after three rather than four years of premed. This was possible, so long as a student completed all of the required courses in that period of time, achieved a sufficiently high grade point, and scored well on his or her Medical College Aptitude Test (MCAT). After three years of premed, when the letter from the medical school came, I was so anxious I could feel my heart pounding in my chest. I do not think I have ever been as full of anxiety as I was at that moment. Had I not been accepted, I would, of course, have completed my fourth year of premed and reapplied; however, that early acceptance saved me several thousand dollars of debt, and for that I was truly grateful.

Lesson 1:
Medical School Starts a Lifetime of Learning

Entrance into medical school in 1964 was no small achievement. In addition to requiring a grade point average that favored As over Bs, the MCAT score needed to be high as well. In addition to having a good personal interview, it was necessary to write an autobiographical sketch of some ten or more pages. It was intended to demonstrate the kind of character the admissions committee considered desirable. Some of the friendships I acquired during those four years remained for a lifetime, despite significant geographic distances. My best man and one of the groomsmen in our wedding party were both medical school classmates, and we continue to remain in close contact, now almost fifty years since we first met.

The adjustment to medical school was more difficult than I had expected. While medical schools were only accepting about one person for every three to five applicants, I did not appreciate the caliber of the students being accepted. The realization of how hard it was going to be to end up in the top 10 percent of such a group sent me into a blue funk. When I began to express my misgivings about my decision to go to medical school, my anatomy professor, Otto Mortenson, sat down with me for a long time and talked to me about his son, who had once gone through the same kind of crisis. He eventually helped me get some professional counseling that assisted me through this difficult transition and allowed me to succeed throughout the remainder of my four years of medical school.

In our first year, when we took anatomy, Professor Mortenson assigned four students to a tank containing a human cadaver that we dissected during the course of the semester. We developed trust and teamwork, which was essential to accomplish the multiple assignments given to every group. After each dissection assignment, the professor tested us orally as a group of four. Before we could proceed to the next assignment, the dissection had to be properly completed and we had to pass the oral questions as a group. There was a subtle competition among the groups, but by the end of the semester, no single group finished more than a day or two ahead of the others. Some students developed anxiety during the first semester, including tension headaches, bladder and abdominal cramps, and even diarrhea.

One unfortunate student was several years older than the majority of us because he had been a high school Latin teacher before deciding to go back to college and apply for medical school. He had a gastrointestinal disorder known as ulcerative colitis, of which most of us in the class were unaware. Ulcerative colitis, like Crohn's disease in the small bowel, is an inflammatory bowel syndrome thought to be partly genetic and partly environmental. Midway through the semester, his condition began to worsen, to the point where he was admitted to the hospital through the emergency room with severe abdominal pain and bloating. The doctors diagnosed him with toxic megacolon, a dreaded complication of ulcerative colitis. This is often associated with perforation of the bowel, which results in the leaking of its bacteria-laden contents into the abdominal space, and is associated with excessive bleeding at times. The condition is considered a surgical emergency, and it frequently requires removal of part or all of the colon. He was taken to surgery shortly after admission to the hospital, and, since he was a medical student, I am certain that the most capable of the university surgeons and gastroenterologists were called in to provide his care. Unfortunately, he did not survive. We learned of his death the next day during our anatomy lab session; the room that day was very quiet and subdued. Ordinarily we filled the room with animated conversations, but that was not the case on this somber day.

During the first two years in medical school, we primarily had basic science courses like anatomy, histology, physiology, pathology, biochemistry, and so forth. The only patient-related course we had was physical diagnosis. Various specialists lectured us and brought in patients on stretchers or in wheelchairs to demonstrate some of the techniques in obtaining a history and examining patients. Wearing our short white coats and armed with stethoscopes, otoscopes, and reflex hammers, we were allowed to examine patients in the hospital.

Five or more medical students had examined many of the patients who were in the hospital each day. At that time, average hospital stays were ten or more days. It required considerable patience on the part of a patient who was being examined by forty to fifty medical students during a single hospital admission. The first patient I ever examined was a woman who had rheumatic heart disease involving a faulty valve in her heart known as the mitral valve. When I went to her room, I could tell she was not interested in having me there. She seemed depressed and sullen. I remember her having difficulty making eye contact with me. I decided that the best approach was to see if I could get her history and examine her. I explained to her that I was aware she must be exhausted and exasperated by having to serve as a teaching tool for so many medical students. I told her that if I were in her place, I would also be sick and tired of being a guinea pig. Then I said that this was the same way that the famous doctors who were caring for her had been trained. I told her that without patient cooperation, there would not be very many good doctors. I do not recall what else I said, but she finally agreed to let me go ahead. She had a classic cardiac murmur because of her mitral valve insufficiency, and I cannot remember ever hearing one so well. She turned out to be a valuable learning experience for me, one that I carried with me during the rest of my years in medical school, internship, and residency.

We had the summers off between our first, second, and third years of medical school. Once the third year started, there was no summer break before we started the fourth year. Many students, including me, could not wait to get into our clinical years. After the second year, a few of us were fortunate enough to get summer jobs in Madison working for doctors in private practice. We were actually paid a stipend for doing histories and physical exams and for assisting or observing procedures in and out of the operating and delivery room over several weeks. We referred to these jobs as externships.

I was fortunate to find an externship at St. Joseph's Hospital in Pontiac, Michigan, not far from Detroit. The externship at St. Joseph's Hospital was a marvelous program that consisted of three weeks of pediatrics, obstetrics, and general surgery. Two other externs besides me were medical students from Wayne State Medical School in Detroit. We became good friends, and they even took me to the Detroit Receiving Hospital, which is where all the charity or indigent patients go for their medical care. They told me it was going to be a zoo, and they were right. The halls had patient gurneys lined up with people who needed knife wounds repaired, gunshots wounds examined, as well as a potpourri of other trauma. Any medical student who wanted to learn to repair wounds was welcomed here, as the number of patients that required care overwhelmed the staff interns and residents.

During my time at St. Joseph's Hospital, I delivered about a half-dozen newborns under the capable supervision of the attending physician. This was six more than I delivered while on my obstetrics rotation during my last year of medical school. The top general surgeon at St. Joseph Hospital, Dr. Larson, was one of the most skilled surgeons (besides Dean Clinic's Dr. Richard Botham) I was ever exposed to. He was careful, decisive, and very dexterous. He wasted little time doing what needed to be done, which also resulted in shorter operating times. This, in turn, helped reduce infection rates, as the longer a wound was open, the greater the opportunity for bacteria to enter it. As a point of interest, air filtration and air circulation systems present in today's operating rooms have helped reduce airborne organisms, so length of procedure doesn't play as much of a role anymore. In addition to the air systems, the prophylactic use of antibiotics to reduce infections for many procedures is very common, particularly for those that involve putting in foreign bodies like GORE-TEX vascular grafts, metals, plastics, and ceramic components in total knees and hips, and so on.

My last two years of medical school were the most enjoyable. Like many medical students, I experienced what is referred to as medical student's disease. What happens, particularly when a student has good teachers in a particular clinical area of medicine, is that the student becomes certain that this is the field to pursue as a career. At different times throughout school, a student will want to become a psychiatrist, pediatrician, internist, cardiologist, surgeon, and so forth. My goal of becoming a research scientist waned once I realized I was more suited for working with people rather than in a laboratory. By the time I started my internship on the George Washington University Medical Service at the DC General Hospital in Washington DC, I had narrowed it down to three: pediatrics, surgery, and orthopedics.

During our senior year of medical school, we each spent three months in a clinical preceptorship that required us to spend time in a one-on-one relationship with someone selected for us in internal medicine, pediatrics, or general surgery. Their practice locations were throughout Wisconsin. My preceptorship was in Milwaukee with a warm and caring internist, Dr. Einar Daniels. It was my responsibility to do a history and physical exam on each of his admissions to the hospital, discuss the cases with him, and write orders for their evaluation and care. I would do this after going over what the orders should be with him first, much like an internship.

I slept in the intern/resident quarters of what was then the Milwaukee Lutheran Hospital. Making rounds with Dr. Daniels gave me an opportunity to see how doctors in private practice interacted with one another. I especially enjoyed the time we spent in the radiology department discussing the findings on X-rays with the radiologists who were all keen on teaching a neophyte like me what the shadows on some of the films represented. Fortunately, the radiology department at the university taught us well so that they were somewhat impressed with what I already knew. Those radiologists gave me an open invitation to come over to the department any time to look over their shoulders as they read and dictated the findings on the hospital X-rays.

Learning to read X-rays was not only important in my internship but also during my residency. UW residents were allowed to moonlight as ER doctors no more than three days a month in private emergency rooms. An ER doctor who could distinguish normal from abnormal on an X-ray saved a number of on-call private practice doctors from having to come to the hospital unnecessarily.

Like most people who know exactly where they were at the time of the assassination, I will forever remember that it was at Milwaukee Lutheran Hospital that I first learned President John F. Kennedy had been shot. I remember being in the X-ray department when I heard the news that was spreading like wildfire throughout the hospital. I went immediately to the interns'/residents' quarters to find a television to follow what was happening. I was glued to the set for several hours and still remember the horrible feeling I had when it was announced that he had died of his wounds.

During the presidential campaign some three years earlier, Kennedy had come to speak on the University of Wisconsin campus. The auditorium in Music Hall was the site for his speech. I got there about a half hour before the speech, and every seat in the place was filled. Fortunately, the people in charge allowed many of us to sit up on the stage, within fifteen feet or so from the speakers' rostrum. Kennedy was as handsome in person as in his photos, and his stump speech was as inspiring as his writings. The memory of being that close to him has become as indelible as that fatal day that was to follow in 1964. His death, as it was for so many others he had touched, made me feel as though a family member or dear friend had just died.

About seven days after graduation from medical school, I exchanged vows with Barbara Ann Werth at St. Paul's University Chapel. We have been married forty-three years, which I am certain would have come as a surprise to my mother-in-law's close friend and also to her older sister, Alice Pahl. Her friend, Mrs. Wheeler, had been married to a doctor who divorced her for a younger woman. She warned Barb's mother, Dorothy, of the same probable fate for her daughter. Alice, childless and known as Al by her friends, was married to Patrick Pahl, a successful tire company owner, who was called Pat. It took me awhile to figure out their genders, particularly since Dorothy had seven other sisters and one brother. This created a long list of names and faces to remember; they were all married, and most had children of their own. Al did not want Barbara to marry me because I was Italian and Catholic. I suppose in her mind that made me less than a prize catch.

Today I think that story is amusing. Al lived to be ninety-five and decided about a month before she died that she wanted to be baptized. Apparently, she had decided it was not worth taking any chances. My wife, Barb, visited her often in the nursing home where she lived for less than a year before she died. I never had the nerve to ask her if she regretted the advice she had given to Barb's mother.

My choices of internship were confined only to acute medical centers, which included Charity Hospital in New Orleans, Boston City Hospital, LA County Hospital, and the DC General Hospital. I thought they would complement the complex-care training I had received as a student at the UW medical school and hospitals, where we saw chronic diseases and bizarre conditions in mostly white people, rather than acute and everyday sorts of problems in more than one race. Because two of my interests were surgical in nature, I decided to pick a mixed medical internship, consisting of nine months of internal medicine, a month of emergency room care, a month of pediatrics, and a month of surgery.

Shortly after we were married, my real-world introduction to internship came as I drove our wedding present from Barb's parents, a 1964 Plymouth Valiant, into the parking lot of the interns'/residents' quarters. There, sitting in one of the parking spaces, was a car on concrete blocks that had all four tires stolen from it. The DC General Hospital was next to the DC jail, so it should have come as no surprise that this might happen in a town noted for its murder and crime rate. Colleagues told me there had been a riot at the DC jail the previous year, and most of the injured inmates had been treated at the nearby hospital.

Fortunately, Washington did not have any race riots during the year of my internship, but one of my medical school classmates and wedding groomsmen, Chang Sup Shim, had his life threatened by the family of a patient who died on a neurosurgery service at the Philadelphia General Hospital. He had been on the service only a few days and was assigned to the care of that patient, along with the resident who had performed the surgery. After the patient died from a severe head injury, Chang Sup found himself followed home by angry family members of the patient, yelling expletives and threatening him. He ended up moving to another part of town and spending nights at the hospital for several weeks to avoid any further contact. It was 1964, and there had been serious race riots in Philadelphia over several well-publicized allegations of police brutality.

The quarters Barb and I occupied in the intern/resident's building consisted of two rooms separated by the bathroom. One room was a living room with rather Spartan furniture, and the other was a bedroom with the equivalent of a double bed and a couple of dressers. The walls were painted cinder block, and it looked very institutional. Each floor had eight similar units and a single kitchen on each floor with an oven, a stove with two electric burners, and a refrigerator shared by everyone on each floor. We used an electric frying pan in our apartment for some of our meals and had to label everything we owned in the kitchen to keep other people from using it. Most of the time, only one other couple really competed with us for the kitchen, and they were from Colombia, South America.

My wife's first Thanksgiving turkey was cooked in our electric frying pan with a large cover. It took forever to cook at low heat and ended up looking like a huge, naked, and blanched bird. Barb did not have anywhere near the experience with cooking that I had acquired during my youth and medical school years. But I didn't have the time to cook, since I was working sixty to seventy hours or more a week with call every third night, which meant only an hour or two of sleep on those nights. I do not know how Barb survived that year with me, as the day after my call night I would crawl into bed right after dinner. Fortunately, she kept busy with her work as a physical therapist, and she loved her job and the people she was working with.

It was an interesting time to be in Washington DC. We were able to see President Lyndon Johnson and Hubert Humphrey escorted from the Capitol into black limos for a parade. During the year I served my internship, we visited all of the national museums and monuments and cemeteries. We took trips to Mount Vernon to see George Washington's estate and gardens. We visited historic Williamsburg and got a feel for what it must have been like living in America at that time. We also went to Gettysburg, Pennsylvania, to see the site of one of the costliest battles in terms of casualties of the Civil War. All of our forays took place on weekends.

We learned what it felt like to be in the minority. Barb, my wife, did her grocery shopping at a supermarket a few blocks from the hospital. Not infrequently, she would be the only white customer in the store.

One night when I was on call, I came home shortly after midnight after having admitted several patients to the George Washington University medical service. I was extremely tired and lay down with my clothes still on next to my wife, who was already sleeping. The bedroom had two single beds with a small end table and a lamp between the two. We had put the end table to one side to push the beds together so we could be close to each other. The phone was on my side of the bed, and I had not checked it in the dark when I had come to bed. A couple of hours later I heard a pounding on our door. When I got to the door with my wife, who was in her pajamas, a large security guard was standing there. He said that one of the nurses had been trying to call me for the past half hour, and she thought I must have taken the phone off the hook. I went back into the bedroom, and the phone was indeed off the hook. But how that happened neither of us could remember. I frequently called Barb from the hospital to tell her that I would be late so that she could go to bed without me. That is probably when it happened. After calling the nurse, I found it necessary to go back to the hospital to see a patient who was not doing well. I do not remember returning home until five or six in the evening the next day, when I finally had dinner and crashed in bed.

Those experiences were physically and mentally demanding. I have a feeling that marriages between an intern and a nonmedical spouse suffered more from this kind of stressful situation. Some quarters of medicine considered this as intern and resident abuse. It certainly tested a couple's ability to weather the meaning of "for better or worse" when it came to their marital vows.

One of my fellow interns, who had graduated from a medical school in a northeastern state, had studied classical guitar for ten or more years. On a couple of occasions, when the interns and their wives got together, he would perform for us. My background in music as cornet and trumpet player gave me a great appreciation of this man's talent. I kept wondering to myself why he had not chosen that as his profession. I later learned that he had decided halfway through our grueling internship to put his medical career on hold and study in Spain under a renowned guitarist. Years later, whenever I hear a classic guitarist, I think about those special nights, preciously few, when he entertained us.

For one month of my mixed medical internship, I was assigned to the George Washington University Hospital instead of DC General. Most of the patients there were upper middle class or higher, in contrast to the indigent patients at the General. All of the physicians there were internists and internal medicine subspecialists. One of the doctors I worked with was a rheumatologist who treated several severely disabled patients. The patients required corticosteroids, quinine, and gold shots—treatments that have been phased out largely over the years by more effective drugs with lower toxicity profiles. I learned from him that at one point in the history of treating patients with arthritis someone discovered that a certain industrial solvent (dimethylsulfoxone, or DMSO), which could be bought in any hardware store, was very effective in relieving joint pain when it was rubbed into the skin over the joint. The mechanism of action on the pain receptors in and around the joints was poorly understood, but it was not long before reports started coming out that patients who had been using this form of treatment were becoming blind. The rheumatologist admitted even using it on a few of his patients before medical literature reported this serious side effect.

The truism I later learned from my orthopedic mentor, Dr. Herman Wirka, about not being the first or necessarily the last to use a new medical or surgical intervention proved to be true. The best example of that has been the use of the drug thalidomide, which doctors used to treat depression. Women who became pregnant while taking the drug stood a significant chance of having a child born without upper or lower limbs or both, a condition referred to as phocomelia in the medical literature. The drug had been used extensively in Germany and had barely been introduced into this country before it was taken off the market. Interestingly, thalidomide has now been shown to have some benefit in killing cancer cells of certain tumors, so it has been allowed back on the market for this specific use only—and with the admonition it not be used in women who could potentially become pregnant while on the medication.

One of the patients I did a workup on at GW Hospital was admitted for the umpteenth time for anorexia nervosa. She looked like someone out of a German concentration camp, and we had to feed her intravenously and with a nasogastric tube to nourish her body. It appeared to me that she was trying to kill herself. I am not certain how much was known about the disease in 1964, but it was certainly one of the forerunners of the eating disorders now so prevalent in girls and young women these days in the United States.

Exposure to leading clinicians in the Washington DC area was one of the highlights of my internship. Several of us interns attended the cardiology conferences given at Georgetown University. Georgetown's Dr. W. Proctor Harvey was a world-renowned cardiologist who had one of the strongest departments in the country at the time. The conference room was equipped with earphones at every desk in the cardiology auditorium where the DC cardiology conference was held monthly. These earphones allowed everyone to hear the subtle sounds of a great number of cardiac arrhythmias and murmurs. Many times, Dr. Harvey would have everyone listen to the heart sounds of one of his cardiac patients. Then he would ask one of the men or women taking a cardiology fellowship at Georgetown what they were hearing and what it represented. After getting their description of the sound and their diagnosis, he would delve into the treatments available for the condition at the time. Dr. Harvey was not only an expert in his field; he was also an enormously compassionate human being. One night while he was entertaining company, he went to the hospital after receiving a call that one of his patients had died. John F. Stapleton, a professor of medicine at Georgetown and Harvey's first cardiology fellow, asked him why he had gone at that hour of the night when his patient had already died. Dr. Harvey had indicated that was when the family needed him the most. This world would certainly be different if all physicians emulated this wonderful person! Many do, but I believe more should.

Other notables who came to teach us directly at the DC General were physicians and scientists working at the National Institutes of Health (NIH). We would select an interesting or complicated case to present to them, and they would use that particular case to base their discussion about the particular disease and the challenges it presented to those diagnosing and treating it. The visiting experts usually knew all of the latest information on the management of particular diseases, and we tried to pick cases that involved their own area of special interest. These were bright and enthusiastic people, and we looked forward to hearing from them.

I spent one of the months of my internship on the surgical service in which the residents supervised the activities of the interns. Since I was only going to be on the service for a month, the residents and staff did not give me many opportunities to do much other than holding retractors and closing wounds, which was understandable to me. I worked very hard on becoming adept at tying surgical knots and repairing the several layers of surgical wounds. There were usually six to eight cases scheduled for a day, and we went from early morning to early evening. We made rounds as a group on our post-op patients and divided the admission workups between us before we went home.

One evening when I had gotten home from a long day in the operating room, I realized that I did not have my wedding ring on. I suddenly remembered putting it in the back pocket of the blue scrub suit I had been wearing. The doctors place all the scrub suits in a large hamper in the doctors' locker room, so I high-tailed it back to the hospital, only to find that the hamper had already been taken to the laundry room. With my heart pounding, I went to the basement to enter the laundry room where there were a half-dozen hampers filled with scrub suits and gowns. Fortunately, one of the first hampers I went through contained the scrubs I had been wearing.

Lesson 2:
Orthopedic Residency Is More
Than an Apprenticeship

Still not sure whether I should pick pediatrics, surgery, or orthopedics, I decided to apply for residency in all three areas, thinking that if one or more programs decided not to accept me my decision would be easier. I was, however, accepted to all three programs. Fortunately, the orthopedic department chairperson at the University of Wisconsin, Dr. Herman Wirka, required me to make my decision within a week, forcing me to come to terms in a hurry. My wife of less than a year, Barb, who had completed her University of Wisconsin physical therapy program two years before, helped me choose orthopedic surgery. She reminded me of my involvement in sports, and my interest in putting broken things back together. The fact that a good deal of orthopedics involved the pediatric age group helped in my decision.

Once I made the decision, I needed to decide whether to risk being drafted into the military during the middle of my residency or to make a commitment to a particular branch of the military to ensure I would enter military service as a fully trained specialist, responsible only for problems in my specialty. The Armed Services had a deferment program called the Berry Plan that allowed for just that option. I applied for the Air Force's Berry Plan and was accepted. It was a relief going into my residency knowing the remainder of my training would be uninterrupted. As it turned out, one of the senior residents at UW had completed three quarters of his training before the Army drafted him. He spent time in Vietnam and had to return to finish another year of orthopedic training after two years in the Army.

I started orthopedic training in July of 1965, excited to learn and develop the skills that interested me. Many of the orthopedic and reconstructive procedures that were developed because of the polio epidemics of the forties and fifties were seldom being performed, thanks to the Salk vaccine. There still was evidence of that part of orthopedic history in the children's hospital, where iron lung machines could still be found in some of the storage rooms. With the advent of penicillin and newer antibiotics, the orthopedic wards filled with patients who had bone infections and whose wounds, treated at times with maggots, had gone by the wayside. It was interesting to hear the older staff talk about the problems they would have with flies as a result of this relatively primitive but effective form of treatment. The ten- to twelve-bed hospital wards also disappeared, in favor of individual isolation, two-bed, and private rooms. It was only after I retired and worked in the Bugando Hospital in Mwanza, Tanzania, that I once again saw the large wards of ten or more beds in each room.

The beauty of my training program was that it not only involved teaching by full-time academic physicians at the five-hundred-bed University Hospital but also allowed us to rotate through two of the three private hospitals as residents. There we were supervised by orthopedic surgeons who had trained at the Mayo Clinic, Cleveland Clinic, University of Michigan, University of Minnesota, and on and on, thereby giving us less of an inbred education. It became evident that while the basic principles and procedures involved in the diagnosis and treatment were the same in all training programs, there were regional philosophies that often dominated thought in some centers or parts of the country. An example was the treatment of clubfeet. Most orthopedists would initiate treatment with corrective plaster casts changed frequently and then perform surgery to correct the residual deformity. Orthopedists in other locations would stay with casts almost indefinitely. Similarly, in patients with congenital dislocation of the hips, surgeons in some areas persisted with traction and cast treatment for much longer than in other areas, where surgeons practiced surgical correction early.

Of course, future long-term follow-up studies eventually showed what the most advantageous treatment was in a given circumstance as far as the patients were concerned. Orthopedic surgeons to this day are dependent on long-term follow-up studies to learn if what they are doing is the best option for their patients. This is referred to as evidence-based medicine. Today's most popular procedure or prosthesis may turn out to be something that doctors abandon later on based on long-term follow-up studies. One of the things that Dr. Herman Wirka taught us about our continual process of learning was never be the first or the last to try a new product. I found that advice very helpful. For example, when the first generation of resurfacing total hip replacements came out in the late 1980s, it was later shown that these implants started failing within five years. I waited until a large number of total hip replacements were being done at the Mayo Clinic before I started using this particular type of prosthesis on my patients. As a result, the number I ended up putting in patients were limited to a few dozen, rather than a hundred or more for those who joined the cause right away.

In 1964, the University of Wisconsin's orthopedic residency was a four-year program that had been accepting three individuals each year for a total of twelve residents at a time. The program must have been stuck on the letter P, as my group consisted of Plotkin, Peterson, and Pellegrino. The first year of the program had us spending about half of our time on surgical fields related to many of the things an orthopedic surgeon has to deal with, including anesthesia, neurosurgery, plastic surgery, and general surgery services.

A residency is similar to the apprenticeships that tradesmen like plumbers and cabinetmakers have, in which they spend a great deal of time learning their fields from on-the-job experience. There were weekly conferences in which the residents researched the subject matter in the orthopedic literature and used that information for their presentations. We were required to attend three weekly meetings. They included a hand conference, children's conference, and a basic science conference where we would meet with clinical associate professor Dr. Peter Golden at a laboratory in the UW medical school. The lab contained a cadaver on which we did various dissections to demonstrate the various surgical approaches or techniques to get us to the anatomic area we would be performing surgery on during our residency and careers.

Dr. Golden had completed his orthopedic training at the Mayo Clinic and had come to Madison to start a solo private practice. He was very interested in teaching and had taken some additional training in hand surgery. He was one of the most principled men I have ever met, and the following stand he took was a perfect example of it. He always felt that the size of a surgeon's practice should be based on how skilled he was in the operating room, in addition to how well he related to his patients and the referring doctors. He was well aware of the need to keep them informed and up to date with his management of their patients. However, he did not approve of the custom of fee splitting, which most general practitioners in Madison required for their referrals. This is different from a family doctor assisting on a case and submitting a surgical assistant's fee to the patient or his insurance company.

After a year or so in practice, he notified his referring doctors that the practice of fee splitting was no longer acceptable to him and that he was going to stop doing it. He felt this was not in the best interests of the patients. I think most people can readily see how this could be abused. In reaction, the majority of general practitioners simply stopped sending him patients. This undoubtedly resulted in a significant loss of income, but he stood his ground. It took several years before some of them referred to him again, and he had to depend on patient referrals and referrals from other specialists to maintain a reasonable practice and income. Fee splitting was eventually determined to be an unethical practice by most medical societies. Unfortunately, while he was in the prime of his practice years, he was slowly becoming blind from a condition called keratoconus, a progressive condition in which the cornea thins and changes shape. He was able to operate for a few years with special glasses, but eventually the glasses failed to give him sufficient correction to allow him to do surgery. As a result, he began to dedicate more and more time to teaching orthopedic residents at the university. His stories about the experts he had trained under at the Mayo Clinic were always fascinating. More important, Dr. Golden's ability to correlate basic biomechanics and surgical anatomy to orthopedics was invaluable.

Our basic science meetings were held in the evenings from six until eight or nine o'clock. The residents also had to present a talk about a basic science or clinical subject. I recall spending a great deal of time in preparation for my first presentation, which was titled "Physical Therapy of the Rheumatoid Hand." Dr. Golden was so impressed he told me I should put it together with a bibliography and submit it to the *Wisconsin Medical Journal,* which is a monthly journal produced by the Wisconsin State Medical Society. To my utter amazement, they accepted it for publication, and I subsequently got several requests for reprints from as far away as Canada. That success spurred my later interest in doing a comparative study of bicycle- and motorcycle-accident victims who were treated at the university hospital. This same journal accepted the study for publication. The chair of the orthopedic department asked me to present my study results to both the Wisconsin State Orthopedic Society annual meeting as well as the state Surgical Society meeting. I think the chair of the orthopedic department offered me a job on his staff based on both of those publications and the job I did as chief resident in my last year.

One of the residents I became closest to was Dr. Kim Lulloff. We were on several services together and bonded with our common interests in sports, our newly started families, and excelling in our chosen field. Kim was a year ahead of me in training and very helpful in warning me about the peculiarities of various orthopedic surgeons I would be meeting. One such surgeon was our pediatric orthopedic surgeon, Dr. Henry Okagaki, who was an excellent surgeon and a warm person, once you were able to get through the hard-crusted demeanor that made the parents of his patients quite nervous at times. He was not a man of many words, and when he did speak, you always hoped he was in a good rather than sour mood. He would give a resident many opportunities to perform a large part of each operation if the resident demonstrated he was a good first assistant. To be a good first assistant you have to anticipate what the surgeon's next move is going to be and make certain you are helping rather than hindering him. Dr. Okagaki recognized this kind of anticipation was evidence the assistant knew the steps of the operation and could therefore perform it when given the opportunity.

He had a large number of patients with scoliosis, which is an s-like curvature of the spine, and these patients often required time-consuming procedures to correct the deformity. A special table was designed for the application of corrective scoliosis casts that allowed us to put traction on the spine while the cast was being applied. Rods with hooks that helped to straighten out the spine had been introduced only a few years before I started my training, and they were a major advance in the surgical treatment of this awful disorder. The other alternative for mild cases was a brace developed by the world-renowned pediatric orthopedic surgeon Dr. Walter Blount, who was humble enough to name his brace after his practice area, Milwaukee, instead of himself, as so many surgeons are in the habit of doing. The Milwaukee brace continues to be part of the conservative treatment of scoliosis. Because of the polio epidemics, orthopedic surgeons got considerable experience with scoliosis, as muscle paralysis produced large numbers of these patients who needed help.

One Sunday afternoon, my wife and I got a call from Dr. Okagaki, who wanted to know if we were going to be home for the rest of the afternoon. Without saying why he was asking, he hung up. About an hour later, he showed up with his camera and a satchel full of camera lenses to take pictures of our six-week-old firstborn, Mark. His hobby was photography, and the pictures he took of Mark are as good as any professional ones. They still hang on the wall in our bedroom. He had that special smile that he often had when he was really enjoying what he was doing, and we looked on in amazement at his generosity. We developed a special bond from that day on, and I owe him a lot for what he taught me in the operating room, especially when it came to being comfortable doing spine surgery.

During my last year of residency, there was a major pediatric orthopedic conference in San Francisco, and he asked me if I would be interested in attending it with him. I certainly could not refuse, and we had a wonderful trip. I not only learned the latest in his specialty but he also treated me to dinner in Chinatown, where he insisted on ordering for me. I think he wanted more authentic food than what the restaurant usually served to tourists. It was a memorable experience.

Of all the surgical procedures that I participated in while I was a resident, one stands out because of its horrific nature. The patient was a twenty-one-year-old woman who came in with a foul-smelling draining area of a bone infection that involved the upper end of her right femur, hip, and pelvis. It had been draining since she was about ten. She had been diagnosed with bone cancer at the upper end of the right femur at that time, and the tumor was treated with massive doses of radiation. This resulted in the destruction of not only the tumor but also the tissue surrounding it, including skin. While the radiation cured her of the cancer, the damage to the other tissues resulted in a serious infection of the bones and surrounding soft tissues.

After several years of antibiotics failed to eradicate the infection, her doctors had advised the parents that the only way to free her from the malodorous drainage and disability was an amputation. The parents refused, so she waited until she was twenty-one and independent to ask for it to be done. The procedure required in her case was a hemipelvectomy. This procedure involves not only removing the entire lower extremity at the hip, but also half of the pelvis.

The pelvis is an area through which major blood vessels and nerves pass, and bleeding is a major concern. The patient was on Dr. Wirka's service, and Kim Lulloff and I were assigned to do her surgery as third- and fourth-year residents. Kim and I had not seen such a case, and, while I did not ask, I do not think Dr. Wirka had seen or done more than one or two in his entire career of nearly forty years. We both studied the technique in our standard text, *Campbell's Operative Orthopedics*, and went to the anatomy lab to check the area out on our cadaver. Isolating the draining area from the surgical incision and staying out of the infected tissue took some careful planning on our part. Kim and I worked as a team, each taking responsibility for major parts of the procedure.

There was a bit of a hum in the surgical halls about our case. During the three hours it took us to complete the procedure, several members of the staff and residents stuck their heads in the room to see how we were doing. The patient survived and did extremely well, considering the nature of surgery we performed. Remarkably, her wound healed without any sign of infection, and when she left the hospital, she was walking with crutches. She was eventually fitted with her prosthesis and learned to ambulate without any assistance. A couple of years later while I was in the Air Force, I learned that she had gotten pregnant and was actually able to deliver her child vaginally.

During that same year that Kim and I had done the hemipelvectomy, Dr. Wirka got an urgent call from the Marshfield Clinic (located about seventy miles north of Madison) asking if he could spare a senior resident from his program for two weeks. The Marshfield Clinic is a regional medical center that had three orthopedic surgeons at that time. Two had been at the clinic just under two years and were taking two weeks off to take their board certification oral and written exams; the third surgeon was recovering from a recent heart attack. The latter surgeon was seeing patients two days a week but doing no surgery, so they were going to be without an operating orthopedic surgeon for two weeks.

Dr. Wirka decided he could not allow one resident to help for two weeks but offered to let Kim and me each spend a week. They gladly accepted. It was agreed that the only surgery we would do during that period would be emergency surgery, but we did see patients in their offices. Most of the patients they scheduled for us were follow-up patients who needed sutures removed or a checkup on the progress of their nonoperative treatments. We saw several patients for the first time at the clinic, but not as many as I expected. The only emergency I had to take care of was an alcoholic who fell asleep outside when the temperatures were hovering around freezing and had severe frostbite and gangrene of several fingers, which needed amputation. In return for our services, the Marshfield Clinic paid each of us five hundred dollars, which I used to buy a new washer and dryer that we used for the next ten years.

Of the nine residents who had been in the program longer than Peterson, Plotkin, and I had, two were foreign-born. One was from Iran, where he had completed his medical training and had come to this country to find an internship and residency. He took his internship in a Chicago hospital before coming to Madison and apparently came from a wealthy family that had reportedly paid twenty-five thousand dollars to some bureaucrat in Iran to get him out of his military obligation. The other resident was born and trained in the Philippines and took his internship in the United States before being accepted into the UW residency program.

Neither stood out as far as the teaching staff was concerned but managed to get through the program by not demonstrating incompetence as physicians. They were able to communicate reasonably well and never irritated the nursing or operating room staff with personality quirks, as some American-born residents did on occasion. Unfortunately, during their rotations through the private hospitals, neither performed much surgery other than wound closures, so their skills were lacking in some of the more complex procedures done at the time.

The Middleton Veterans Administration (VA) Hospital was one place where both of them would have many opportunities to get experience and acquire those skills. Residents, under the watchful eye of Dr. Sion Rogers, were doing almost all of the procedures. When I was a senior student in medical school rotating at the VA hospital on the orthopedic service, Dr. Rogers's teaching and personality helped influence my decision to pick orthopedic surgery as a career.

Before coming to the Middleton VA Hospital, Dr. Rogers had been in private practice in Madison and, in fact, would trade call with Dr. Golden, who was his good friend. During the course of his career, Dr. Rogers had developed a duodenal ulcer that had required surgery. He eventually decided to leave the stresses of private practice to come to the VA as their full-time orthopedic surgeon. He was responsible for teaching the UW medical students and residents clinical orthopedics, as the VA hospital had become one of the many medical-school teaching sites in Madison.

Two cases involving one of the residents proved that even outside of private practice Dr. Rogers could not avoid stress. One such example occurred while he was teaching the Filipino resident how to remove a disk fragment from beneath a nerve root emanating from the spine. The surgeon must carefully dissect and tease the disk fragment from the nerve root to avoid damage to it. This can be extremely tedious because of the amount of inflammation and scarring that develops in the area of the ruptured disk. The most satisfying part of the procedure is to see the tension on the nerve root release after removing the disk fragment. The removal of the disk fragment involves the use of an instrument that has alligatorlike jaws, specifically designed for the task and the disk fragment frequently comes out as a single, large oysterlike fragment. Dr. Rogers had apparently gotten the resident to do the dissection appropriately but he did not realize that the resident was mistaking the nerve root for the disk fragment. When Dr. Rogers asked him to remove it, the instrument grabbed the nerve root. Instead of pulling out something that looked like an oyster out came a long spaghettilike structure before Dr. Rogers could say, "Stop!"

Dr. Rogers's pleas were too late. The resident had removed the nerve fibers. He looked up at the resident and the anesthesiologist and told them to hold everything as it was. He left the operating room and said he would be right back. With his cap and surgical gown still on, he took the elevator to the cafeteria, bought two pints of milk, apparently to coat his now-stressed stomach, and came back to complete the operation for the resident after he changed back into a sterile gown and gloves.

What was remarkable was that, other than a small patch of numbness, the patient had no additional pain or loss of motor (muscle) function. I suspect Dr. Rogers must have felt his prayers were answered, given the lack of significant patient disability from this mishap.

The other incident occurred when Dr. Rogers and the same resident were treating a patient with a displaced fracture in the middle of the patient's forearm. He had elected to have the resident use a rod rather than a plate to secure the fractured bone. The rod, which is referred to as an intramedullary rod, goes into the center of the bone, which is hollow except for marrow or fat. The plate goes onto the surface of the bone; held there by a number of screws. In the process of introducing the rod into the bone, the resident got the rod stuck about halfway in. The instrument we use to put the rod in can also be used to extract it by using a hammer and hitting a platform on the introducer but in the opposite direction. Occasionally it is necessary to attach vise-grip pliers to the introducer to have a larger area to pound on.

After failing for forty-five minutes in his attempt to back the rod out of the bone and using every expletive he knew, Dr. Rogers told the anesthetist to quit because he had exhausted his vocabulary. He closed the surgical site and covered the incision with sterile dressings with the end of the rod sticking out. Dr. Rodgers connected the rod to a rope, pulley, and weights for traction, and eventually it came out several days later. He told the patient what had happened and that once the rod was out they would fix it with a plate and screws. To the best of my knowledge, the fracture ended up healing and the patient was satisfied. I am not certain how many pints of milk or Tums Dr. Rogers took following this case.

I should make it clear that as a teacher of surgeons it is difficult to know what is in the mind of an inexperienced surgical resident who may be doing a procedure for the first time. Mistaking a nerve root for a disk fragment and inserting an intramedullary rod into a bone and not knowing when not to pound it in further when it is first does not progress into the bone are things that Dr. Rogers had little control over. Unfortunately, acquiring experience as a surgeon—as occurs in many other fields—comes with making mistakes. Since then, there have been significant advances in teaching surgical techniques. Surgical technique laboratories for specialized procedure have been developed throughout the country, and are run by surgeons with considerable skill and ability to teach.

One of the most disappointing experiences I had as a resident occurred when Dr. James Huffer and I were removing part of the joint of our adult patient's scapula (shoulder blade) because she had been diagnosed with a malignant tumor called a sarcoma. In this particular case, it was Dr. Huffer's decision that, because the shoulder socket itself was part of the scapula, we should perform a forequarter amputation, since the scapula and the arm were included in the removal. The patient would have a functionless extremity if we just removed the scapula. Dr.

Huffer felt she would likely have better function with a prosthesis than a limb that hung uselessly at her side.

She had had a breast malignancy about twenty-five years previously. In addition to a mastectomy, she had received radiation treatments to the site of her surgery. Apparently, it had been done when the radiation beams could not be controlled as they are now. At this time it is possible to focus the radiation precisely so that the depth and location of the beams is limited primarily to the site treated, and there is very little scatter to surrounding normal tissues. A small number of patients some twenty or more years later develop malignancies in the areas exposed to wide and heavier doses of radiation used at that time. She was one such example, as her scapula was directly behind the breast that had been irradiated.

Our patient was being used as a teaching case for two medical students spending a month on the anesthesia service. The process of anesthetizing patients with a general anesthetic involves first starting intravenous fluids through a needle placed in an arm vein, next administering a sedative through the intravenous channel, and then administering a gaseous anesthetic through a mask over the face or through a tube passed into the trachea (windpipe). The tube, referred to as an endotracheal tube, has a deflated balloon that prevents gas from escaping. Once the tube has been placed and the balloon inflated, the tube is connected to an automatic ventilator that expands the lungs with oxygen and the gas.

One of the critical measures in placing the tube is not to go beyond the trachea into one of the air channels. The way to prove that the tube has not gone too far is to listen with a stethoscope to both sides of the chest to make certain you can hear the breath sounds on both sides. Unfortunately, the anesthetist allowed the medical student to introduce the endotracheal tube in our patient and listen to the lungs. The anesthetist either did not check the lungs or made the same mistake the medical student did, because after an hour or so into the procedure the patient's blood pressure started falling for no apparent reason.

The anesthesiologist had left the operating room a number of times during the procedure, with the medical student in control of the head of table. The anesthetist drew blood from the patient when he was having difficulty figuring out what was happening. We stopped operating and packed the wound with large cotton sponges. They were temporarily able to raise the blood pressure with medications called vasopressors, but, after a while, this failed, and the patient went into a cardiac arrest, failed to respond to electroshock treatments, and died on the operating table. The blood test results came back shortly after the patient died and showed findings consistent with severe metabolic acidosis (disturbance in the body's acid-base balance, resulting in excessive acidity of the blood).

A postmortem examination revealed that she had had a left endobronchial intubation (the tube had passed beyond the trachea into the left air channel), resulting in the lung on the right side of the chest not being ventilated or getting any oxygen. This resulted in low oxygen and high carbon dioxide in the bloodstream, accounting for her metabolic acidosis and death. Universities are teaching centers by definition; however, those responsible for their care should never put patient safety in jeopardy. This was one lesson that was hard for me to learn, as I agonized over the loss of that patient for weeks. I would have loved to have been at the UW anesthesia department's monthly conference when they reviewed this complication and death. This particular conference is referred to as the morbidity/mortality conference. If honesty had prevailed, there had to have been some red faces after discussing how this case might have been handled differently.

Lesson 3:
Military Medicine Is Different from Civilian Medicine

My assignment in the Air Force was Sheppard Air Force Base, an Air Training Command (ATC) base in Wichita Falls, Texas, frequently the hottest spot in the nation in midsummer.

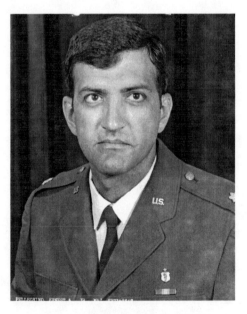

Figure 1 USAF Major Ernie Pellegrino

The base not only served as a training area for many of the technical fields, but it was also where pilots from Germany were trained on our fighter planes. The adjacent communities had a significant retired military population so that part of what we did involved medical and surgical care for these men and their families.

After my basic military training of six weeks was over, my orthopedic practice in the Air Force resembled in large part what my civilian practice in Wisconsin was going to be like.

When I entered the Air Force, my wife and I already had two children ages three and one and a half years old. Because I was the father of two children, the Air Force did not assign me to one of the few Air Force hospitals in Vietnam. The military often sent seriously injured Air Force personnel to a regional medical center in Ramstein, Germany, or to Wilford Hall Medical Center in San Antonio, Texas.

The Sheppard AFB Hospital was a regional center with a 325-bed capacity. The hospital commander, a colonel, and the orthopedic department chair, a lieutenant colonel, "Dr. Bones," were career officers. Dr. Bones was only about two years older than I was. The remainder of the department included "Dr. Brooks," who had only completed his first year in orthopedics and who had also just completed the first of his two-year military obligation; Dr. Robert Fitzgerald, a general medical officer; and finally an orthopedic surgeon, "Dr. Maurice Mansfield." Dr. Mansfield had reportedly completed an orthopedic residency at Georgetown University Hospital in Washington DC. After the first few months, I was asked to serve as acting chair whenever Dr. Bones was on leave or unavailable.

Dr. Mansfield was single and had the personality of a used-car salesman trying his hardest to get you to like him. Early on, we became friends, and I invited him for dinner a few times with my wife and young family. Initially, I did not play a role in evaluating Dr. Mansfield's judgment or skills, as this was the responsibility of Dr. Bones, the career officer and chair of our department. In addition, Dr. Mansfield and I were supposedly equals, as we had just completed our residencies before joining the Air Force. I recall Dr. Bones scrubbing (participating or actively observing another surgeon performing an operative procedure) on only a case or two of mine initially, and I suspect it was not many more times for the other fully trained doctors before they were given free rein in the operating room. To my surprise, Dr. Brooks, with less than half of his residency completed, went for the most part unsupervised. The exceptions were if he asked someone to assist or instruct him in a procedure he was not comfortable doing without help. Fortunately, most of the time he used good judgment in the year that I supervised him at his request on the more complex cases he had scheduled for surgery.

As we approached the eleventh month of my first year at Sheppard Air Force Base Hospital, it became apparent there had been an inordinate number of complications occurring in the patients that Dr. Mansfield was treating. This became apparent to me on a weekend call in which it was the responsibility of the on-call doctor to make hospital rounds on all patients on the orthopedic service. I became particularly concerned when I saw a fifteen-year-old girl who supposedly had a routine removal of plate and screws done by Dr. Mansfield that resulted in her hip being broken. Normally I wouldn't have gone to the trouble of pulling and reviewing the whole file of X-rays on someone else's patient, but seeing this patient suffering from what should have been a simple procedure piqued my curiosity.

What I discovered upon reviewing the X-ray file as well as the old medical records was that at age four or five she had originally had the plate and screws inserted into the upper end of the femur. The plate and screws had been used to hold together the bone in her hip to improve stability, which at that time had the residuals of a congenital hip dislocation, a condition usually noted at birth. This procedure, called a femoral osteotomy, is common in the practice of a busy pediatric orthopedic specialist in a metropolitan area. The plate and screws, called "hardware," are usually removed about a year after the procedure. Otherwise, the remodeling of the bone that occurs after several years in a child will eventually bury the hardware in the femur so that it can no longer be identified on the surface. Her X-rays, taken before the disastrous procedure performed by Dr. Mansfield, showed that the plate had indeed become centralized within the bone and that the hardware could not have been the source of any of her symptoms. What was causing her to have symptoms was that at fifteen years of age she was developing degenerative or arthritic changes that went unrecognized by Dr. Mansfield.

This patient ended up getting me started on a crusade that ultimately resulted in several more months of collecting information and documentation on a level of incompetence that should never have been tolerated in the Air Force, or anywhere else for that matter. I was upset about what I had discovered and decided to speak with Dr. Bones about this case and a number of others I had begun to document. I was disappointed when he responded by asking me to calm down. He indicated that he did not believe in making any waves and reassured me that in a year Dr. Mansfield would be out of the Air Force and the problem would go away. I could not believe what I was hearing but assumed that he wanted to avoid having one less orthopedic surgeon on the call schedule and the increased patient and surgical load for the remainder of us. He also indicated that when Dr. Brooks and Dr. Fitzgerald finished in a month, a fully trained orthopedist and another general medical officer would replace them.

I decided to send a letter to Dr. G. W. Hyatt, professor and chairman of the division of orthopedic surgery at Georgetown University Hospital, since he had been the last person responsible for Dr. Mansfield's training. In this letter I did not enumerate the specifics of the dozen or more cases that I had documented but simply indicated that Mansfield had been having an unusual number of complications and making poor judgments and that I wanted to know if he could help me understand this situation better. His reply indicated that Dr. Mansfield had only spent one year in the Georgetown orthopedic program, coming there from Indianapolis with excellent recommendations from Dr. Carl Martz. Dr. Hyatt said it had become evident that this so-called fourth year for finishing was not fulfilling Dr. Mansfield's needs. He informed Dr. Mansfield that he needed two, three, and possibly more years of training before he could be considered competent. Dr. Hyatt indicated that his errors in judgment had been substantial. He indicated it was his intent to give him one year of further training and that if his problems remained insoluble, to drop him for potential certification. Dr. Hyatt ended by saying that he not only questioned his competency as an orthopedist but his basic competency as a physician.

I should mention for the reader that I confronted Dr. Mansfield after I received the letter from Dr. Hyatt regarding his need for more training. Dr. Mansfield told me that Dr. Hyatt informed him of this a couple of months before he was to have completed his fourth and final year of residency. He admitted he had been accepted as a resident to the Sinai Hospital orthopedic surgery program in New York City after he had graduated from one of the schools of osteopathy, which in general have lower admission standards than medical schools.

After his first year at Sinai Hospital, he spent the second year at a children's hospital in Cleveland and then returned to Sinai for his third year, where he was dropped from the program upon the completion of that year. He was able to get a surgeon from Cleveland to write a letter of recommendation for him to get into the Georgetown program. Dr. Mansfield indicated that he had told the Air Force that his last residency director had advised him he would need at least one more year of residency before the director would agree to make him board eligible. Mansfield asked if he could take that year of training while in service and if the year could come out of his Berry Plan obligation. The military denied his request. I suspect that it was because they had no one to fill in for him at Sheppard or that they did not think it was their responsibility to do this without his making a commitment to repay each year of training. To this day, it is not clear to me how far up the chain of command this information and request actually reached. At any rate, no one at Sheppard was aware of his circumstances until I received a reply from Dr. Hyatt.

After I received this response from Dr. Hyatt, I did a retrospective evaluation of all the charts of Dr. Mansfield's patients since he started at Sheppard. I felt obligated to document how dangerous it was to have him continue to serve as an unsupervised fully trained orthopedic surgeon. I had to do this during off-hours, and it took months to accomplish because my patient load had become significantly higher when it became evident that we not only had a problem surgeon but also an incompletely trained surgeon as well; Dr. Brooks was doing more than he had been trained to do. It was also during this period of time I had to study for my board certification oral and written exams, requiring me to put the chart review on hold for a number of weeks until I passed both of those exams.

Before my orthopedic board exams, I was making weekend hospital rounds on all our patients when I noticed one of Dr. Brooks's patients looked jaundiced. I asked an internist, Dr. James Rose, to see the patient. Dr. Brooks had done lumbar disk surgery on the patient unsupervised two days before. After he examined the patient and did various tests, including an electrocardiogram, he told me he was going to have to treat the patient for high-output cardiac failure, a condition he had a hard time explaining, especially in such a young person.

I remembered from my medical school and internship training that high-output failure frequently is the result of an abnormal pathway between an artery and a vein. This occurs when blood moves directly from an artery into a vein, and can be caused either by a congenital or iatrogenic (doctor-caused) connection between an artery and a vein. This abnormal pathway results in an increase in the volume of blood returning to the heart because it has avoided a large volume of capillary beds. The capillary system slows down the flow of blood to the heart, resulting in a normal blood flow. When the blood is shunted, the heart has to work much harder; a normal heart will eventually fatigue and show signs of failure, as it did in this patient.

I was well aware that one of the serious complications of lumbar disk surgery is a vascular injury. An instrument known as a pituitary rongeur can cause the injury. The instrument looks like a small bird's beak on the end of a long metal rod, which is manipulated by a scissorlike grip. The surgeon uses the beak to grab hold of the disk fragments and pull them out from under the nerve root, thereby relieving the pressure on the nerve, which has produced the leg pain commonly associated with a ruptured disk. When a surgeon pushes this instrument too far into the disk, it may come out the other side of the vertebra and remove a piece of a major blood vessel wall. Since the major arteries and veins coming from the abdominal aorta and vena cava are right next to each other, it is possible for a piece of the artery and vein to be simultaneously removed, so that the artery can now flow into the vein, creating a passageway or shunt known as an arterio-venous fistula. A doctor makes the diagnosis by listening with a stethoscope to the groin area or lower abdomen over the femoral artery. I heard a machinery type of murmur similar to a harsh swishing sound corresponding to patient's pulse. It was exactly what I expected, and I immediately called a vascular surgeon who confirmed my findings and corrected the problem by repairing the defects in the blood vessels.

The patient did well after his vascular procedure, and his cardiac status returned to normal. He was lucky, as this same type of vessel injury, had it not resulted in a fistula (abnormal pathway), could have just as easily resulted in his bleeding to death in the operating room. A surgeon performing an open lumbar disk operation has to be aware that this is a cause of a sudden drop of blood pressure during the course of the removal of disk material with a pituitary rongeur. It is extremely unlikely that a physician with one year of orthopedic training would have been aware of this reason for the sudden loss of blood pressure. This case would be a gold mine for a trial attorney should it have happened in civilian practice. However, in the military, particularly in 1970, there would have been little opportunity to sue the government and one of its military employees.

When I had completed my review of the cases I had collected regarding Dr. Mansfield's incompetence, I formally wrote them up to once again approach Dr. Bones and now also the hospital commander in an effort to stop the potential further harm that might befall those patients coming under Dr. Mansfield's care. The evidence was overwhelming, and the final action was satisfying, although it occurred later in Dr. Mansfield's two-year obligation than I had originally hoped. Because of my investigation, our superiors removed Dr. Mansfield from the orthopedic service, and we became responsible for taking care of the remainder of his patients. Dr. Mansfield's remaining time as a physician was confined to working in the dispensary as a general medical officer, seeing patients with colds, flu, earaches, and so on. There he never saw another scalpel, except with those few patients who came in with minor lacerations that he could repair with a few stitches in the dispensary.

While I was happy with the result, the long process it took to accomplish it embittered me. I was also disappointed with the supervision of partially trained personnel. After mulling it over for a few weeks, I finally decided to do something that might rectify a system that would allow for something like this to happen. After discovering that the U.S. Air Force Surgeon General was Lt. Gen. Alonzo A. Towner, I decided to write him a letter. I explained who I was and what I had done to document a series of surgical catastrophes and misjudgments by Dr.

Mansfield. The list was lengthy. He had cut a nerve root while performing a lumbar disk surgery and lied to the patient as to what happened. He had broken a patient's tibia in the process of removing hardware used years previously and had broken a young girl's femur in an attempt to remove a plate used years ago, while failing to realize it was buried within the bone and not the source of her pain. He had failed to utilize X-ray in the operating room, resulting in doing an operation on the wrong bone and a second operation. Moreover, he had unknowingly cut a tendon during bunion surgery and failed to recognize a fractured femur that was not healed enough to allow a patient to be taken out of traction, resulting in refracture.

I told the surgeon general that the tragedy of this situation was that the chief of the department was aware of Mansfield's incompetence and failed to adequately supervise and initiate remedial action in a timely fashion. The hospital commander and the chief of personnel were aware of several of the problems and had failed to make changes. I indicated that it was not until January 1971 after my continued prodding that the chief of the department had finally made a copy of my list of disastrous cases and submitted them along with my letter from Dr. G. W. Hyatt to the hospital commander. I pointed out that it was nearly nineteen months before Dr. Mansfield was relieved of his orthopedic responsibilities.

The other issue I addressed in my letter was the supervision of Dr. Brooks, who was assigned to the orthopedic service from June 1968 to June 1970. I pointed out that Captain Brooks had one year of internship and one year of orthopedic residency for a total of two years' experience beyond medical school compared to the minimum of five years for the fully trained orthopedist. I indicated he had apparently been able to convince the chief of the department that he had considerable knowledge and competence, since in his last eighteen months on the orthopedic service he had been allowed to take night and weekend call without any supervision. A review of the orthopedic records revealed that in his last eighteen months he performed approximately 293 elective operations, of which approximately 238 were unsupervised, which is almost unheard of for a partially trained surgeon. I listed a number of his cases that were misdiagnosed or had complications related to inexperience. The most egregious one was a patient who had two normal cartilages removed from his knee because the doctor missed a bone tumor in the femur close to the knee, which I later discovered as the source of the patient's pain. In fairness, I pointed out that errors in judgment and complications, albeit uncommon, occur even in fully trained experienced surgeons. Dr. Brooks, however, denied his patients the opportunity to have such a surgeon give them his or her opinion.

I pointed out that while it might appear that I was trying to embarrass the department chair and commander, I was mainly concerned about the military process that allowed this to happen. My purpose was to raise awareness with the following questions and suggestions:

- What efforts are made to discover the true competence and completeness of training of so-called specialists prior to entrance into the service?

- When an individual with a service commitment is found to be incompetent or incompletely trained prior to entrance into the service, what efforts are made to further his training or provide responsible supervision?

- After a surgeon is found to be incompetent while in the service, how long and how many patients must it take to correct the situation?

- Is it wise to take a physician fresh out of a residency and make him assume the responsibilities of chief of a department in one of the Air Force's busiest regional hospitals, and, if so, what objective tests or criteria are used to that decision?

- Should any individual with less than half of his surgical training completed ever be allowed to assume full responsibility for the emergency and operative management of patients in an essentially peacetime military setting?

Finally, I indicated that I was very interested in General Towner's opinions and was hopeful that my questions might help initiate or better clarify policies dealing with the military surgeon and his patients.

The reply to my letter to the Air Force surgeon general came a week or so after I mailed it. I was somewhat surprised as well as disappointed at its content. Lt. General Thomas H. Crouch, an orthopedic surgeon and deputy surgeon general, wrote the letter to me. His explained the service's dependence on records they receive but admitted, "There is no means whereby we can examine every incoming doctor individually but must rely on his records and the comments of his supervisors." He went on in his reply to try to give justification for the system that was in place, which I obviously thought was broken, and made a concluding statement that raised the hair on the back of my neck: "In comparison with civilian practice, I can truthfully state that our practice of medicine in the Armed Forces is clearly superior."

What bothered me most about this response was that it represented a very defensive stance and did not address all of my concerns. I decided to respond with a letter that expressed my disappointment and suggested that I might take my concerns to the next level. I told him that Major Mansfield had informed me he had notified the Air Force of his status prior to his entrance into the service and that the military had denied his efforts to secure further training while in the service. In addition to incorrectly classifying Major Mansfield as fully trained, I pointed out that no one had notified his hospital commander and supervisors of his status. I also pointed out my concerns regarding partially trained specialists assuming full responsibility for emergency and operative management of patients in an essentially peacetime setting had gone unanswered.

I pointed out that our experiences with the practice of medicine in civilian life were dissimilar, as I had not yet seen the quality of medicine referred to in my original letter in any civilian hospital of comparable size and staffing during my training. Finally, I pointed out that if those who practice medicine in the military consider these circumstances acceptable, then perhaps our legislature should be given an opportunity to make a judgment as to whether this is the form of health care the public should have in the future.

All during this time my wife, who in addition to looking after our first two children was pregnant with our third and last child, was concerned that someone was going tell my superiors what I was up to and they were going to stop me by sending me to Vietnam. When she finally went into labor, she waited a bit too long to ask me to take her to the hospital. Upon our arrival at the hospital, the obstetrics nurse checked her progress and yelled, "Dr. Pellegrino, get some scrubs on so you can deliver this baby!" Fortunately, it was almost a straightforward delivery. The obstetrician managed to get there a few minutes after my baby boy, Todd, arrived. He relieved me of having to deliver the placenta and repair the episiotomy (small incision made to enlarge the vaginal opening) I performed to prevent a recurrence of a third-degree vaginal tear she had the misfortune of having during the delivery of our first child, Mark.

Fortunately, my wife was wrong. A few days after I mailed my response to Major General Crouch, he replied, addressing me curiously as Dr. Pellegrino rather than Major Pellegrino. He apologized for giving me the impression that he was trying to gloss over the issues I brought up. He admitted they had gone into the background of my allegations and found them to be entirely factual; investigated the handling of the situation and found it to be unsatisfactory; and were indeed working on an improved procedure for assessing the exact professional capabilities of incoming physicians prior to their reporting date. In closing, he said, "I hope you can take it on faith that the situation you brought to our attention was most unusual, that we are alarmed by it, and that we sparing no effort to prevent its recurrence."

This last letter from General Crouch responded in a more specific way to my concerns, seemed to result in some position changes, and was much more satisfying to me personally. I was aware at the time that the complimentary remarks contained in it as well as the Air Force Commendation Medal I was awarded at the completion of my tour of duty were intended to produce that same effect. Even to this day, I harbor some resentment that it took so long and so much of my time to accomplish what the career officer in charge of the department should have done when I first brought it to his attention.

To the best of my knowledge, Dr. Mansfield left the Air Force and got a job working in the emergency room and outpatient service of a metropolitan hospital somewhere in California. I do not know whether he completed the requirements necessary to become board eligible in orthopedic surgery. One thing I am certain of is that he has never been admitted to the American Academy of Orthopedic Surgeons. The academy requires all candidates not only be board certified but that they have at least two members of the Academy recommend them and not have any members opposed to their membership for good reasons. I have looked for years for his name on the bulletin of people making application but have never seen it.

Dr. Mansfield certainly is the most egregious example of incompetence that I have ever been exposed to in both the military and in civilian practice. However, I do remember several years ago reading in one of the national news magazines about a cardiac surgeon who went from civilian practice to the military and had a high death rate that ended up being the result of incompetence that had been hidden from the military before he made it his career. It would appear from this latter example that the system in the military still needs to be tuned up. In defense of the military, whatever system is out there to filter out incompetence is only as good as the information it receives from outside sources. There is potential danger when someone uses personal references from individuals who are good friends and who do not really have true insight into their problems. These problems can also be buried in some medical records room, not accessible to the person making a positive recommendation. Unfortunately, more problems are likely to occur until someone brings a record of disasters to the attention of a person or committee responsible for peer review.

It was not until the 1950s and 1960s that hospitals became more aware of the need to establish physician committees to review medical records, morbidity (complications), and mortalities. It was not until departments met on a regular basis that they discussed these issues together. It was even more important to have a separate committee review and discuss individual cases compiled by trained personnel in the medical records area.

The committee often sent letters to physicians, asking them to explain circumstances that looked suspicious. If a response was not forthcoming or appropriate, the committee would ask the physician to appear before them to answer questions regarding a complication or course of action. If the committee felt that explanations or answers were not satisfactory, then they would conduct a retrospective review of all of the surgeon's operations of a certain kind or occasionally all of his or her cases to determine if a pattern had been developing. At a minimum, the surgeon might be put on notice, asked to have a second opinion on a particular kind of scheduled procedure, or asked to have a second surgeon present during the surgery. At the maximum, his privilege to perform a given procedure or even all of his privileges might be removed until he has obtained further training.

Drug or alcohol abuse might be a reason for a surgeon's problems, and, if the committee found that to be the case, they would require a rehabilitation program during the removal of privileges. After a successful rehab program, the committee might then restore privileges, followed by a period of supervision and random urine or blood tests. A second recurrence after restoration of privileges would likely result in expulsion from the hospital staff.

Lesson 4:
Power without Ethics Is an
Incurable Problem

My practice began with a solo orthopedic surgeon, "Dr. Bruce Blair", for whom I have great respect. We elected to provide orthopedic coverage for East Madison Clinic (EMC), a multispecialty group of twenty-plus doctors who had no orthopedic surgeon. Because Dr. Blair had his own office and personnel in another location, it fell upon me to provide three quarters of the EMC's orthopedic coverage. I developed a very busy practice in a short period and elected to join the clinic at the end of my first full year, something Dr. Blair was not prepared to do at the time and never did. We continued covering each other's practice on weekends until a few years later when he joined a group of three other orthopedic surgeons who practiced mainly at Madison General, rather than St. Mary's Hospital where the majority of my practice was located. I ended up taking my own calls weekdays and on weekends. When I was not in town, doctors at the Dean Clinic, the largest multispecialty group in town with a three-person orthopedic department, followed my patients.

In the three years at the East Madison Clinic, my practice grew too large for me to handle alone. I asked the clinic to recruit a second person. I interviewed two strong candidates who respected me, my practice, and liked the city of Madison; but both decided not to join my practice because the clinic's salary offer was not competitive with the salary and benefits others had made. Reluctantly, I found it necessary to give the EMC notice of my resignation. I could no longer stay because my long hours and frequency of being on call, night and day, were having a deleterious effect on my family life.

Later I received a job offer to join a practice in Portland, Oregon, with an orthopedic surgeon who had taken his residency at the University of Wisconsin. I was seriously considering moving, thereby leaving the community where my wife had spent most of her life. She was relieved when, unexpectedly, the Dean Clinic asked me to join their orthopedic department, which I gladly accepted. I was not eager to leave this beautiful, intellectually stimulating area, my patients, and my professional associates.

I wanted to retain my position as a clinical instructor to the University of Wisconsin, teaching orthopedic residents who all had three-month rotations at St. Mary's Hospital. I loved the opportunity to do clinical studies and over the years made three presentations of the results of my clinical research. I presented my results at the annual Wisconsin State Orthopedic Society meetings and had one poster exhibit at the annual meeting of the American Academy of Orthopedic Surgeons in Las Vegas, Nevada, and Anaheim, California, respectively.

The first person I remember as an example of an unethical surgeon in private practice was neurosurgeon "Dr. Henrique Seeker." Dr. Seeker practiced at all three private hospitals but primarily at Madison General, where he had been chief of staff and where all of his problems had been documented. As a resident, I vividly recall being the second assistant in an operation in which a staff orthopedic surgeon at St. Mary's Hospital had asked Dr. Seeker for his participation. I remember thinking at the time that he was a capable surgeon; however, I had a different opinion of him as a person. I had overheard a conversation he was having with another staff surgeon in the doctors' locker room as the surgeons were changing back into their street clothes. The staff surgeon was mentioning how many requests he had received in the mail for donations from various charitable organizations now that the year was ending. Dr. Seeker's reply was that he never gave them a damned cent and they usually stopped asking after a few years. I have since been told that Dr Seeker would pledge a great deal of money for some fund drives to gain a favorable public impression and then never pay it.

When it came to income, Dr. Seeker outstripped his competition by as much as five or six times. One of his former associates indicated that in the early 1960s he was booking (dollars billed) five hundred thousand dollars in fees compared to eighty thousand dollars for the next-busiest neurosurgeon in their group. Whenever he had a patient without insurance who happened to be a farmer, he would have the farmer sign the deed to the farm over to him as collateral. According to a former chief of staff at Madison General Hospital, Dr. Seeker eventually ended up owning one of the larger hog farm operations in the state; something he thought ironic for someone whose religion was opposed to eating pork.

In his book *We Are All Pink on the Inside*, Dr. James F. McIntosh wrote that Dr. Seeker was the most respected neurosurgeon in southern Wisconsin in 1967. He was chief of staff and had the biggest practice at Madison General. The utilization committee at Madison General did not have as high a regard of him after they found several disturbing cases that warranted a thorough investigation. With

Dr. Seeker's knowledge and initial approval, the executive committee chose a special review committee.

The committee spent one year reviewing his practice. They contacted two prominent neurosurgeons from out of state to review these cases and interview Dr. Seeker. In 1968, the final report of the review committee included a recommendation that Dr. Seeker's privileges be revoked. Before taking action, the executive committee held a special session to enable Dr. Seeker to refute the charges.

The major charge involved performing unnecessary surgery, reporting procedures not performed, and making inaccurate reports (made public by the local press in 1971). The executive committee of the Madison General medical staff held a second special hearing a month later with Dr. Seeker and, following that hearing, the committee recommended voluntary resignation, reapplication in three years, and further training. The committee offered the doctor an opportunity to present his defense to the medical staff, but he declined. He asked instead to present his case to the hospital board. In January 1969, after an extensive interview, the board of directors of the hospital dismissed him.

While I had finished my orthopedic residency on June 30, 1969, I obviously did not have any firsthand knowledge of what was taking place at Madison General Hospital. In the course of my practice I learned about a number of incidents that I felt were profoundly unethical that involved Dr. Seeker. After letting this dark history of medicine lay dormant in my mind for more than thirty-five years, I decided to talk to a number of physicians who I thought would have firsthand knowledge of the cases used against Dr. Seeker. The case that Dr. John McClung, an excellent anesthesiologist, called the trip wire that caused Dr. Seeker to come tumbling down from the pedestal he had placed himself upon happened to be a patient to whom Dr. McClung had administered general anesthetic. Dr. Seeker was performing a carotid arteriogram, which involves placing a needle into one of the carotid arteries on either side of the neck so that radio-opaque dye can be injected and all the blood vessels of the brain can then be visualized on X-rays. It was used to show the abnormal blood flow that goes to a tumor or a vascular malformation, such as a congenital arterio-venous fistula or an aneurysm, which is a ballooning of a cerebral blood vessel that could rupture at anytime during one's life. Of course, now ultrasound and MRIs have replaced most of the reasons to order a carotid arteriogram.

During the procedure, Dr. Seeker spent an inordinate amount of time trying to get into the patient's carotid artery, which was small because she was a child. Frustrated because of his inability to get into the artery, Dr. Seeker decided to abandon the procedure and told Dr. McClung to awaken the patient. In filling out the anesthesia record, Dr. McClung wrote that the surgeon aborted the carotid arteriogram. The patient eventually left the hospital without having had the arteriogram.

One of Dr. McClung's partners, Dr. David Noll, was doing a routine chart review and discovered that the chart on the young patient with the aborted arteriogram contained a document signed by Dr. Seeker. The document Dr. Seeker had dictated was that the carotid arteriogram had been normal. A search in the X-ray file room revealed no X-ray pictures of a carotid arteriogram present in the patient's X-ray folder. The report dictated and signed by Dr. Seeker had been a complete fabrication.

I remembered Dr. David Noll telling me about a patient with arteriogram evidence of a terminal malignant brain tumor whom Dr. Seeker took to surgery for a craniotomy and brain biopsy. The procedure involves making a large skin flap on a shaved head, removing a variable size piece of the skull bone and then removing a piece of tissue called a biopsy from the tumor site to be examined by a pathologist. Many if not most surgeons get a frozen section done on the specimen before closing the wound in order to be certain one has removed the right tissue, and it also gives a preliminary diagnosis that can be related to family members who are usually anxiously awaiting word from the surgeon. In this particular case, the surgeon made a skin flap, controlled some bleeding vessels, and then, without removing bone and taking tissue, closed the skin flap back up.

The chart on this patient was signed out in the record room as the patient having had a craniotomy and brain biopsy, but no biopsy report was found in the chart. It always bothered me why the anesthesiologist would not question Dr. Seeker about this kind of a practice. I could only assume it was because he was an extremely powerful man, both physically and in the political realm. For example, when and after he had been chief of staff at Madison General Hospital, he would park his big Cadillac in a no-parking zone behind the hospital, and no one from security had the authority or audacity to ticket his vehicle. Physically he was intimidating with dark hair, olive completion, and bushy eyebrows. He reminded me of a human bulldog or Sicilian mafia hit man. I think some people were afraid of what might happen to them if they complained. This is all conjecture on my part but it may explain, but not excuse, those who kept silent about what had apparently been going on for several years.

Recently I was trying to get corroboration of the craniotomy case from "Dr. Sven Erickson," a highly regarded orthopedic surgeon who had been a friend of both Dr. Seeker and Dr. Noll. While Dr. Erickson, who is now in his eighties, did not have a recollection of that particular case, he said there were a number of cervical and lumbar laminectomies that Seeker had done that were simply sham procedures where the skin, fat layer, fascia, and muscles were incised but no lami-nectomy done or tissue removed. A laminectomy is a procedure that involves exposing the back of the spine and removing a variable amount of bone (lamina) to relieve pressure on nerves and to remove disk material or a tumor, which also can compress nerves or the spinal cord. Dr. Erickson's story corroborated the ethics involved in the craniotomy case.

A pediatrician at Madison General also told me about a case that, while not negligence or frank unethical behavior, was one that demonstrated a personality trait on the part of this neurosurgeon that I found very bothersome. This particu-lar case involved a teenage girl who was having problems with her mother and developed a hysterical paralysis. Dr. Seeker had had the patient admitted to the hospital to have a pneumo-encephalogram, which is a painful procedure that involves removing spinal fluid and replacing it with air that is allowed to migrate up into the fluid spaces of the brain. When there is a tumor that occupies space in the brain, it pushes the fluid spaces aside or collapses them, and this change can be seen on the X-ray film once air replaces the fluid.

The hospital protocol required that pediatric residents admit and evaluate pediatric patients. The resident's evaluation discovered that the girl really had a psychosomatic problem related to a mother-daughter relationship and that she was using this pseudoparalysis to get attention. The pediatric service informed Dr. Seeker of what they had found. While Dr. Seeker had not seen or examined the patient, whose family doctor had referred her, he insisted that she have the pneumo-encephalogram because it would "teach her a lesson." Had this been a parent subjecting their child to such pain, she might be arrested for child abuse, but unfortunately the pediatric service was too timid to interfere. The patient ended up enduring an unnecessary and painful procedure, not to say anything about the potential complications that could have occurred from the procedure itself.

As one might imagine a person like Dr. Seeker was not going to take the actions of Madison General Hospital, the executive committee, and the review committee involved in the collection of information lightly. According to Dr. James McIntosh, Dr. Seeker filed a lawsuit in federal court charging that under the Fourteenth Amendment his constitutional right to due process had been vio-lated. A trial was held in 1971. Two years later Federal Judge James Doyle issued a decision stating that although Dr. Seeker's right to due process had been denied, his failure to ask for a hearing before the entire active medical staff barred him from obtaining relief in court. The suits against the individual members of the review committee were dropped a year later, and the U.S. Court of Appeals in

Chicago affirmed Judge Doyle's decision. Please note that this suit was about the legal due process and was not about the medical malfeasance I have described.

Based on the information I have provided here, which came in large part from Dr. McIntosh's book and my interviews, I had a hard time understanding what specifically the hospital had done that denied Seeker his constitutional right to due process. I suppose it is possible that there was something written in the hospital bylaws that was not followed exactly as written, but he was given ample opportunity to defend his indefensible actions.

A weak-kneed Wisconsin State Board of Medical Examiners found Dr. Seeker's professional conduct from 1965 to 1968 unsatisfactory and only served him with a formal reprimand and a vow to monitor his practice for an additional two years. They based this decision on the fact that Dr. Seeker had practiced at Methodist Hospital and several out-of-town hospitals since his dismissal from Madison General. Supposedly, there were no violations at those institutions during that period.

The Dane County Medical Society failed in its attempt to have a civil suit filed by then District Attorney Humphrey J. Lynch to get Seeker's license revoked. The district attorney sat on the request for eighteen months and then withdrew the complaint because he thought it would have a divisive effect on the medical community and that the proceedings would involve a long, drawn-out, and expensive legal battle. I can only surmise that justice did not prevail and that powerful influences behind the scenes played a role in this conclusion. One such influential individual was a judge who was an ex-patient and open supporter of Dr. Seeker.

Dr. Seeker left Madison and Wisconsin to start a practice in the Southwest. According to Dr. Erickson, Madison General Hospital never had any requests for practice information made by any hospitals outside of the state. It is entirely possible that Seeker only put down Methodist Hospital in his references, and they only reported what took place at their institution without volunteering any information about the problems he had at Madison General. When I hear trial attorneys complain about how doctors and the licensing board sometimes fail to expose and discipline bad doctors, this case always comes to mind. In the end, it was the legal profession, and not the medical profession that protected this doctor.

Lesson 5:
Some Doctors Have Problems with Egos, Tempers, and Rigidity

In 1967, the University of Wisconsin's athletic department needed a full-time sports medicine doctor to supervise their medical needs. Up until the sixties, generalists in the student dispensary played a role in the nontraumatic problems in this piecemeal affair. When injured, the youngest staff person in the orthopedic department often treated the athletes. There was an aging trainer and a couple of younger athletic trainers who attended at football games. The coaches and players often relied on him for diagnosis and treatment recommendation for their injuries and referred to the elder trainer as "Doc."

Because the athletic department did not think they had a physician who was truly dedicating his practice to their department, they advertised in journals to find someone to fill an obvious need for that position. They thought the person they chose, a general surgeon interested enough in sports to write a book about sports injuries, was an expert.

Over a period of years, it became abundantly clear that his medical knowledge and training in the musculoskeletal system were spotty at best when compared to a fully trained orthopedic surgeon. This became evident to me as a junior resident in the program when I took care of a patient whose delay in diagnosis resulted in the loss of his limb. He was an African American player for Wisconsin who had been injured in Minneapolis when the Badgers played the Minnesota Gophers. He had been tackled while running with the ball, and his left knee was severely injured, with three of the four major ligaments stabilizing his knee completely torn.

Someone with a sound knowledge of the mechanism of this injury knows that it often takes a force that can dislocate the knee to completely tear the anterior, posterior, and medial collateral ligaments of the knee. The team physician and trainers examined the player on the field. They felt he needed to be hospitalized because of the severity of his pain. They placed his leg in a cast to immobilize the knee in preparation for surgical repair of his ligament injuries when he returned to Madison.

Unfortunately, when a knee dislocates and then goes back in place right away, the true severity of the injury is not appreciated by those not familiar with the mechanism of injury required to produce multiple ligament damage. It is critically important to understand that with the degree of ligament damage this athlete had suffered, a dislocation most probably happened.

Along with the ligament damage, a dislocation can also damage the blood vessels supplying blood to leg. This damage can either be a complete or partial tear of the popliteal artery (major artery located behind the knee). There will be no pulse in the foot in a complete tear, but with a partial tear, there will usually be a pulse until a clot forms at the site of the partial tear and occludes the vessel. The way to recognize this kind of an injury is first to suspect the possibility this could have happened and then to get an arteriogram, which will show whether the blood vessels are normal. Tragically, this was not done.

Because of the cast and the patient's skin color, no one recognized the vascular damage in time to save his leg, which had to be amputated just below the knee. When he was transferred to the university hospital in Madison, I was the resident responsible for the care of his amputation wound, which took a long time to heal, as vascular injuries frequently do.

Because of this case and several much less significant cases that were brought to the attention of the chair of the orthopedic department at University Hospital, the athletic department decided to search for an orthopedic surgeon who had fellowship training in sports medicine. In 1974, they chose "Dr. Manny Brash," who trained in New York under a professional football team physician. Dr. Brash had been serving as the team physician at the Naval Academy in Bethesda, Maryland. He was well respected, knowledgeable, and a skilled surgeon, which appeared to leave him very little room for humility. He dominated conversations, professional or otherwise, and his results (according to him) were always very good or excellent, as average or poor when it came to his surgical feats was not in his vocabulary.

Dr. Brash and I actually became good friends because of our having sons of the same age who played hockey together on an elite traveling team for fourteen- and fifteen-year-olds. Calling Brash's personality a disorder might be a little severe, but you can be the judge. During several of the indoor youth hockey games in which our sons played against local teams, Dr. Brash would stand up against the Plexiglas surrounding the sheet of indoor ice. Most of the parents sat in the stands. He often would get very upset with the referees when they made a call he did not like or did not make a call he thought they should have made. His deep baritone voice could be heard resounding over the Plexiglas and ice arena, so the referees had no trouble hearing him. After a tirade of verbal abuse from Dr. Brash during one of our sons' games, the referee stopped play and asked our boys' coach to ask Dr. Brash to leave the ice arena or he would give the team a five-minute bench penalty, during which time they would have to play shorthanded.

Most of the parents sitting in the bleachers were glad to see the referees take a stand, as Brash's outbursts were an embarrassing display to many of them. What was even more astounding was that a similar episode occurred at Camp Randall Stadium during a Big Ten football game. A Big Ten referee did not like what he was hearing coming from the Badger bench area where Brash, as team physician, was holding court. The referee stopped the game to warn the coaches to stop Brash's outbursts of verbal abuse or the team would be penalized.

Dr. Brash did not take criticism very well. This is best seen in an incident that involved his decision to return UW quarterback Randy Wright to a game in which he suffered a head injury that knocked him unconscious momentarily and amnesic for the remainder of the game. Immediately following the injury, Wright lay on the field motionless for what seemed like an eternity while the trainer Gordon Stoddard and Dr. Brash examined him. A stretcher was brought onto the field to carry him to an ambulance that was parked just outside the gates of the stadium. The ambulance brought Wright to University Hospital, where X-rays were taken and someone from the neurosurgery department saw him. It is not clear whether this was a resident or a staff member.

The neurosurgery department found no skull fracture and his vital signs were stable, so he was allowed to return to the stadium. Standard protocol, when someone has had this kind of a head injury, which has the potential for a late bleed that can be potentially lethal, despite normal X-rays and initial examination, is to bench the player. It is also important to repeatedly examine him and then give him, his family, or his roommate advice about the signs of increased intracranial pressure from bleeding to prevent a potential catastrophe. When Dr. Brash elected to return him to the game and run the risk of further injury, two neurosurgeons in the Milwaukee papers criticized him the next day. Later in the week, I also criticized him, in the form of a letter to the editor in the *Wisconsin State Journal*.

As a team physician for one of the city of Madison public high school football and hockey teams, my criticism was that he had set a bad precedent. I was concerned that high school coaches might now expect team doctors like me to allow them to put their better players back on the field or ice rink after similar injuries.

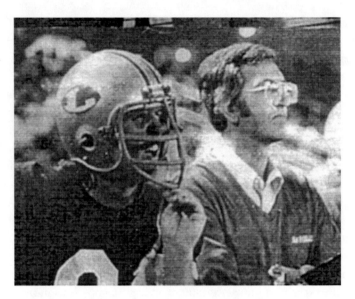

Figure 2 High school team physician

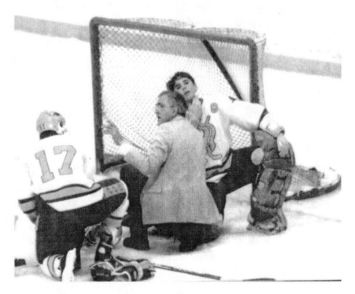

Figure 3 High school hockey team physician

Brash rebutted my criticism in the paper, and while he agreed with my princi-
ple, he did not think I had any business commenting on his treatment because I
was not on the field examining Wright. He was not aware that the UW trainer,

Dennis Helwig, who also went out on to field to examine Wright with Brash, was a good friend of mine. Helwig's mother was a patient of mine, and I had done a successful total knee replacement for her arthritic knee. The trainer told me how spaced out Wright had been after the head injury, and when a radio program interviewed Wright, he could not remember the events of the injury, which supported the fact that he had been knocked unconscious. This type of head injury is called a concussion. Delayed epidural bleeding from small arteries around the brain covering, known as the dura, can occur hours after a head injury causing brain damage, and X-rays at the time of the injury can look normal in these patients.

The Milwaukee neurosurgeons and I all felt observation would avoid further brain damage and risk. Dr. Brash's first wife subsequently told me that she thought we were right, which was a risky admission on her part. She was a friend and lovely woman who often played tennis in a group that included my wife. At the time, I greatly appreciated her confession, as well as the many comments and letters of agreement I received from peers, patients, and people I did not even know. One such person was Dr. Samuel B. Harper, a retired general surgeon who wrote, "Thanks for standing up and being heard. Someone had to do it and I was pleased to see you had done so. One of the less desirable characteristics of society is arrogance which seems to be one element in the whole incident." It is of interest that Randy Wright, who went on to play in the NFL, ended his career because he had had a number of concussions that led him to believe he was at risk of permanent brain damage, particularly in older age. I am confident that the team physicians and neurology consultants he saw for these concussions advised him of this possibility.

Despite our public disagreement, Dr. Brash and I remained friends during his remaining years at the university. Unfortunately, when he eventually decided to leave the university to join a busy sports medicine group in the South, he said several uncomplimentary things about the university and Chancellor Donna Shalala. He essentially burned any bridges of returning to the university, which he may have regretted ten or so years later when he reportedly made some inquiries regarding the availability of positions here and in Minneapolis.

To his credit Brash did popularize a procedure initially developed by others to reconstruct the anterior cruciate ligament (ACL) and has been on the committee of team physicians for the Olympics for many years. Also to his credit was his ability to take responsibility publicly for operating on the wrong foot of a football player who was scheduled to have a bone spur removed from his heel. Dr. Brash slightly tarnished this uncharacteristic act of humility when he stated the wrong side also had a spur, which could have required surgery in the future. Of course, the public is not aware that heel spurs are common, particularly as we age, and most of them do not require surgery because the heel spurs themselves seldom produce pain. More often, it is the fascia (tendonlike tissue) that attaches to the spur or heel bone that gives pain. This is referred to as plantar fasciitis or inflammation of the plantar fascia. In either case, nonoperative treatment often works, making surgery unnecessary.

An interesting fact regarding errors made by university doctors is that all the physicians and surgeons working for University of Wisconsin hospitals are considered state employees and are protected by state statute against malpractice suits unless they are filed within ninety days of the alleged incident. The rest of us in the community, including people like myself with clinical rather than academic appointments, even at the associate professor level, which I had attained, did not have this luxury. This was a sore point among many community physicians, because the cost differential for liability coverage was substantial.

Another university surgeon I became aware of but had no direct contact with was "Dr. Jonah Hale," a man of short stature and a thoracic surgeon who ruled with the proverbial iron fist. He retired about the time I became a medical student. I am certain that medical centers around the country had similar characters, but residents learned early in their training when they rotated on the thoracic service that they did exactly what was expected of them or they suffered the consequences—regardless how inane the expectation might be. Frequently, if you were not doing what was expected of you as an assistant in the operating room, Dr. Hale would use a large surgical instrument to rap your knuckles. He apparently felt you would learn to be a better assistant if he physically punished you.

Dr. Hale also believed that the best way for patients to receive fluids that they could not take by mouth was through a method known as clysis. Clysis consists of using a bottle of the desired fluids connected to intravenous tubing and a needle attached to it that was placed into the patient's abdominal subcutaneous (i.e. fatty) tissues, instead of directly into a vein. This was usually uncomfortable for the patient but depended in part on the type of fluid, rate of flow, and total volume. Eventually this fluid is absorbed into the tissues and makes its way into circulation through the capillaries. Dr. Hale was the only one who insisted in using this antiquated method of fluid delivery at University Hospital.

Fortunately for the patients, the only time clysis was evident was when Dr. Hale made his rounds before going to the operating room. Every morning, well before Dr. Hale arrived on the floor, the residents removed all of the intravenous fluid needles from his patient's veins and inserted them in their abdominal soft tissues with almost no flow. As soon as Dr. Hale finished making rounds and had gone to the operating room, the junior residents or interns would remove the needles from the abdomens and start a new IV on each of his patients. How they were able to sustain that for decades is a remarkable feat in itself, but fear is a great motivator.

Lesson 6:
Incompetence Happens

During the last several years of my private practice and for a few years after I retired in 1998, a number of defense attorneys and Dr. Tom Meyer, who was the director of the University of Wisconsin Medical Extension Center in Madison, WI, called on me to evaluate cases and physicians. I reviewed malpractice claims for the defense attorneys, and they wanted my opinion as to how defensible the doctor's involvement might be. I tried to be as objective as possible, and when I thought it would be best to settle rather than defend the case, I did not hesitate to say so. Occasionally I could sense some disappointment on the part of the attorneys, since the insurance carriers paid them on an hourly basis, and there are not a great number of hours involved when the case is settled.

The physicians evaluated by Dr. Meyer's group of consultants, of which I was one of several, were doctors having an unusual number of complications on the staff of certain hospitals. There were also times when Dr. Meyer was concerned about a surgeon doing procedures he or she was not qualified to do. The UW Medical Extension Center provided this service to hospitals located in as well as outside Wisconsin. The evaluations consisted of reviewing copies of patient hospital records and originals or copies of X-rays. As orthopedic technology has advanced over the last couple of decades, the general orthopedic surgeon cannot possibly keep up with all of the changes in subspecialty areas, such as spine, oncology, hand, pediatric, complex trauma, and complex joint reconstructions. That is not to say that the general orthopedic surgeon could not do straight forward, easier cases, but each individual surgeon needs to be aware of his or her limitations and able to refer patients to a fellowship-trained subspecialist or university center when appropriate. Greed, inflated ego, or both often sway the surgeons, who fail to recognize their limitations and think that having a new product manufacturer's representative in the operating room during a complex case is good medicine.

I evaluated one particular surgeon during this time who stands out among the rest. He was in his late forties. "Dr. Sam Banks" had been in practice for about ten years in a moderate-sized city in Florida. After a period, it became apparent that he was having far too many surgical complications compared to the rest of the orthopedic staff at the hospital. The hospital he was working at decided to review his surgical cases and began to find a large number of concerns. After he was asked to explain some of them before a hospital review committee, he decided to resign from the staff and start a practice in a smaller town in the state of Wyoming. It was at this hospital in Wyoming that some of the same kinds of problems began occurring, and, while he had no peers to review his work there, the hospital executive committee and administration decided to find an outside source that could independently review this surgeon's practice. That was how the UW Medical Extension became involved in his evaluation.

The Extension Center director, Dr. Tom Meyer, decided to ask the individual to submit office charts on twenty patients Banks had done surgery on in the last three months, including the patients the hospital had some concerns about. The doctor also was scheduled to come to Madison and take a standard orthopedic written exam that was to be graded by machine. The Extension Center would discuss the results of the tests with him as part of a personal interview. The doctor agreed to participate in this evaluation so that he would not lose his hospital privileges at the Wyoming hospital.

Dr. Meyer's plan was to use two orthopedic consultants to accomplish this evaluation. He asked Dr. Andrew McBeath, the chair of the Department of Orthopedic Surgery at the UW hospitals and medical school, and me. It was his intention to have me review the outpatient and hospital records and for Dr. McBeath to conduct the personal interview, using the surgeon's answers on the exam as the basis for the interview. Meyer expected both of us to write up a report and recommendations based on the evidence found in the records and responses to the interview.

Unfortunately, between the time we were first asked to undertake this evaluation and the actual time we were to complete it, Dr. McBeath was diagnosed as having an advanced malignancy of cells produced by his bone marrow. Dr. Meyer was unable to find another volunteer from the university to replace Dr. McBeath and asked if I would be willing to do both parts of the evaluation, which I ultimately agreed to do.

The review of the office charts and hospital records was tedious work, and I spent between twenty-five and thirty hours doing it. The office records revealed a number of instances in which Dr. Banks was making diagnoses without having the established criteria necessary to make them. Dr. Banks then proceeded with surgeries that appeared to be unnecessary. The fact that these patients failed to show improvement after having the procedures was evidence of his misdiagnosis. This was even more evident in several cases in which he performed the removal of supposedly torn knee cartilages. Dr. Banks had done these surgeries in the absence of appropriate findings on physical examination and in the absence of diagnostic tests like an arthrogram or MRI. An arthrogram is a relatively low-tech procedure in which dye is injected into the knee, coating the internal structures, such as a meniscus (cartilage pad), and ligaments (joint stabilizers) like the anterior cruciate (ACL) and the posterior cruciate (PCL). A MRI utilizes the effects of a large magnet that is pulsed to change the polarization of the cells of our tissues, producing images that look like the actual structures.

It also became evident from the records that he was doing spine surgery with technology that required more training and experience than he had. Instances of reoperation for complications were clear evidence of his inadequacy.

His test results, which were the basis of the interview, were more surprising than I had anticipated. He had answered more than 50 percent of the questions wrong! My purpose in asking the questions I had was to try to understand his thought process in answering the questions on the test, particularly the ones he got wrong. I did not reveal his test results or tell him whether he had answered the question correctly. The questions on the tests were all multiple choice, and a clinical history with and without lab and X-ray results accompanied each question. In some instances, the question asked what studies should be ordered given the clinical information. My approach to the interview was to ask questions that involved his reasoning in making his decision—why one choice was right and the others wrong on a number of the questions on the exam.

We had allotted approximately two hours with a ten-minute break in the middle for the interview. I hoped my use of a nonconfrontational technique as well as my line of questioning might serve as a learning experience for him. Where there was any controversy as to whether there was more than one right answer, I gave him the benefit of the doubt. However, there were not many such instances. My impression was that the first hour had gone fairly well and that perhaps he was accepting this as a learning experience. When he came back for the second half, it was apparent that I was wrong. When we came to questions that he became aware he had gotten wrong, he was not only unaccepting of the correct answer but also started to become somewhat belligerent. This was no longer a comfortable atmosphere, and I looked forward to it ending. Fortunately, shortly before it ended he calmed down and nothing threatening happened.

When he asked me how well I thought he had done, I told him I was not at liberty to give him any information on his evaluation at that time. I told him that he and the hospital would be getting the complete results of our assessment in a couple of weeks. In my report, I pointed out the number and character of instances in which he deviated from the standard of good orthopedic practice based on the charts and records reviewed. I pointed out how poorly he had done on the examination, and the number of times his explanations fell short of those of a more knowledgeable and competent orthopedic surgeon. I finally described his demeanor during the examination that made me uncomfortable.

When it came to my recommendations, I felt there were some basic procedures, like a carpal tunnel release and routine fracture management, for which he did not need supervision or a second opinion. I made a list of procedures that I did not feel he should be allowed to do without a corroborating opinion from a board-certified orthopedic surgeon. Some procedures required supervision. I felt these restrictions should be in place until he took at least a six-month remedial program in an approved orthopedic residency program. I also said that he needed to take the current *Orthopedic Update* examination. This is available every two to three years and requires reading a five-hundred-plus page book published by the American Academy of Orthopedic Surgery, detailing the new developments in the various areas of our specialty. There is a voluntary examination associated with each issue of the book, and I recommended he take it.

When nonmedical people read this true story of Dr. Banks, they have to wonder how to know whether the doctor they are seeing is substandard. The unfortunate reality is that it is difficult for anyone without access to professional, often confidential, information to know. A neat professional office with impressive-looking diplomas on the wall is not an indicator of an individual's competence and integrity. When it comes to nonemergency, otherwise known as elective, procedures, a surgeon who does not discuss nonsurgical alternatives with his patient in addition to a proposed surgery is one who should raise a red flag in your mind. It is particularly important if the patient has not attempted nonsurgical alternatives prior to seeing the surgeon. Ask the surgeon for all the alternatives and the likelihood of success; this is an important part of the assessment of your surgeon. If she becomes defensive or brushes off alternatives without a believable explanation, this should also raise a warning to the patient.

When she provides you with a convincing and logical explanation of your problem and how surgery may help, seriously consider asking the surgeon if she is opposed to your getting another opinion before going ahead with the procedure. It is always a good idea to ask the surgeon how many of the procedures she has done and what her recommendation would be should the procedure not be successful. If she says that she would refer you to a medical center or to another specialist, perhaps that is where or with whom you should be having the surgery in the first place! In getting a second opinion, go to a medical center with several specialists in the same specialty as the surgeon you originally consulted. Most primary care doctors (i.e., family medicine and internal medicine physicians) would be glad to refer you to wherever you might want to go or might also be a resource of where to get another opinion. However, these doctors may only use one or two other people in that particular specialty, which limits you to only those individuals. Contacting the national specialty organizations is often helpful in getting the names of several reputable individuals within reasonable driving distance.

Lesson 7:
Becoming an Expert Witness Is Uncomfortable but Necessary

"Brenda Young" was a fifteen-year-old patient I inherited from my former associate when he decided not to join the East Madison Clinic (EMC) that had employed both of us as contract orthopedic surgeons. I had decided to become a member of this group because I found that 80 percent of my practice at that time was coming from referrals within the clinic or their affiliates. Because Brenda lived on the east side of Madison, it was much more convenient for her to come and see me at EMC. The patient had gotten to know me briefly as I made rounds on her one weekend when she was in the hospital for a knee operation for a recurring kneecap dislocation. The development of a condition called a compartment syndrome, in which swelling in the muscle compartments results in impaired circulation to the muscles, complicated her post-op course. If someone does not recognize this condition early enough, the muscle cells gradually die and eventually all or most of the muscles in that particular compartment will die. At the time I made hospital rounds on her, I reviewed the chart and had some concerns about the management of her complication. I chose not to say anything to the patient, her parents, or my associate at that time.

A patient with compartment syndrome complains of pain that exceeds what one would expect from surgery or the injury to the extremity. A doctor can recognize this when a patient is not favorably responding to the usual doses of pain medication. Another finding associated with this syndrome is numbness that does not fall within a typical single nerve distribution. Each sensory nerve in the leg has a typical pattern that may be to one side or the other of the leg or foot, front or back, extending down to and including one or more toes. The pattern of numbness seen in a compartment syndrome is called a stocking-glove pattern. In other words, the area of numbness would cover the skin of the leg as though it were in a stocking. Because of the lack of sufficient blood in the muscles of the leg, the muscles begin to lack the ability to function and contract. Therefore, the patient will find it difficult to move the ankle and toes. When a compartment syndrome has started, passive movement of the toes markedly increases the pain in the leg, where the main muscles that move the toes and ankle are housed. Passive movement occurs when the examiner tries to push a patient's toe up or down instead of the patient doing it. Lastly, the leg appears to be swollen and feels tense when palpated by the examiner.

What is critical about this condition is that if the diagnosis is made within the first six to eight hours after its onset, the death of muscles can be prevented. The procedure done to relieve the pressure is known as a fasciotomy. This involves making an incision the length of the leg and cutting the tissue known as fascia, which is the lining or walls of the muscle compartments. When this is done, the muscle will almost explode through the opening created by the fasciotomy. When only some of the diagnostic criteria are met for muscle death, one can further confirm the diagnosis by measuring the pressure within the compartment. A doctor could do this by using equipment present in all hospitals at the time, including an eighteen-gauge needle, a syringe with a three-way stopcock, sterile fluid, and a mercury blood pressure manometer. When the pressure measured in the compartment is forty millimeters of mercury or more, the diagnosis is confirmed. Today there are commercial devices designed to do this task without the above equipment.

Brenda's surgery, called a Hauser procedure, involves the tendon that goes from the kneecap to the leg bone, referred to as the patellar tendon, along with a piece of tibia (leg bone). This tendon is moved about a half inch or so to realign the direction of pull on the kneecap. If done properly, this will prevent the patella from dislocating. Her procedure had been done in the late morning, and by early evening she was complaining of excruciating pain. When the pain medications were not reducing her pain, the nurses called the resident on call.

The resident on call happened to be a general surgery resident rotating at St. Mary's Hospital from the university's general surgery program rather than an orthopedic resident, so his orthopedic knowledge base was minimal. He did come to see the patient and decided that the problem was that her cast, which went from the base of her toes to the upper thigh, was too tight so he split the cast with a single split. Orthopedic residents are taught to split a cast by bivalving it. This involves making a slit on both sides of the cast, but in either case splitting the plaster alone does not relieve the constrictive forces on the extremity. It is necessary to cut through the circumferential padding, known as Webril, all the way down to the skin. Once this is done, a cast-spreader can be inserted into the slit to increase the space for the leg. If a cast has been bivalved, a doctor can actually lift off the top half to inspect the leg and to observe and palpate the presence of leg swelling and tension directly. This was not done. In addition, the resident did not record the presence or absence of numbness or examine her toes by passively moving them to see if that increased her leg pain.

Several hours after the cast had been split, the nurses called the resident again, and he simply ordered an increase in the dose of her pain medication. Between seven and eight in the morning, her surgeon made morning rounds, removed the top half of her cast, examined her leg, and made the diagnosis of compartment syndrome. Instead of putting her on the surgery schedule to have an emergency fasciotomy to prevent further damage, he instead arranged to take her to surgery in the afternoon. This allowed him to see his office patients that morning. Consequently, it was almost eight hours after he had seen her in the morning and at least twenty hours after the onset of the symptoms of her compartment syndrome.

The findings at the time of Brenda's fasciotomy had to have been very alarming to her surgeon. When the surgeon made the incision and exposed the muscles of her lateral compartment, he noted the muscles had already undergone significant necrosis (death) and were already partially liquefied. He was forced to remove a significant amount of dead muscle from both the lateral and anterior compartment of her leg. Her incision was initially left open to allow the swelling to go down and further demarcation of dead versus viable muscle to occur. After a second procedure to remove dead tissue known as a debridement, the surgeon closed the wound. Rather than another cast, Brenda was placed in a removable splint so that the wound could be accessed more easily.

Her surgeon Dr. Bruce Blair followed her for a couple of months until she started seeing me at the recommendation her mother and due to the distance she traveled for her appointments. After several visits in my office, it was apparent that her permanent residuals were going to include a drop-foot– and varus-foot deformity associated with claw toes and numbness. A drop foot is a condition in which a person can no longer voluntarily raise the foot up at the ankle, and a varus foot deformity is one in which the foot turns inward beginning at the middle of the arch. Claw toes are those that do not lie flat and instead appear to be humped. There are orthopedic procedures to help correct these kinds of problems that were developed following the polio epidemics that left thousands of patients with similar deformities caused by muscle paralysis, as opposed in this case to muscle death.

I recommended a tendon transfer using a tendon coming from an unaffected posterior compartment and passing it from the back to the front of the leg between the two bones in her leg (i.e., the tibia and fibula). This tendon was also contributing to her foot deformity, so it was also useful to get rid of that deforming force. I also recommended correcting the foot deformity by fusing the bones on the outside edge of the foot. This procedure is known as a wedge osteotomy and involves making a cut through a bone with a saw or chisel-like instrument. A closing wedge osteotomy involves making two cuts through the bone separated by a specified distance and having the ends of the cuts come together at the same point, thereby creating a wedge of bone, which is removed. Closing this space changes the direction of the remaining bones. This was successful, and she derived significant functional and cosmetic benefit from it. She no longer had to wear a drop foot brace to keep from tripping, and she could now wear shoes.

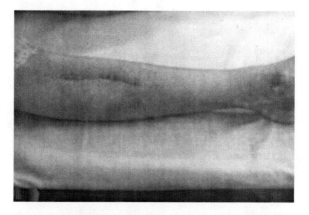

Figure 4 Residuals of leg compartment syndrome: Brenda Young

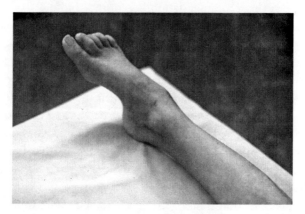

Figure 5 Residuals of leg compartment syndrome: Brenda Young

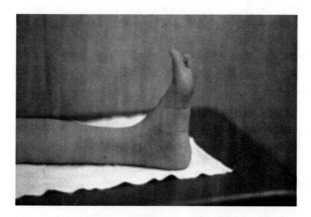

Figure 6 Reconstructed ankle and foot: Brenda Young

During one of several post-op visits, the patient's mother advised me she was seeing a lawyer, Mr. McManus, because she and her daughter were not made aware that these kinds of problems could occur from her original surgery. She was concerned that her daughter's surgery was not done properly. She asked if I would support her in this contention. I told them that in my professional opinion I did not think anything was done wrong to cause her compartment syndrome. However, I did think that the delay in diagnosis and treatment did result in her daughter's disability, which could have been prevented, in large part, with a timely fasciotomy.

Part of the responsibility of an expert witness in a malpractice case is to provide the plaintiff's attorney with your opinion of the quality of the diagnosis and treatment of the patient in question (the plaintiff). It is critical to provide the attorney with as much information on the medical subject as possible. A trial lawyer is trained to organize his or her case in a way that convinces a judge and jury that his or her client has been harmed and deserves compensation. Some attorneys lack basic medical knowledge and depend on you to educate them. I was not aware of this fact until I became involved in this particular case, which was one the first cases in which I testified as an expert witness. I became aware of McManus's weakness in this area after my first conversation with him in my office. I even made an effort to provide him with material he could read to help him. This included an article in the *Journal of Bone and Joint Surgery* that had been published before Brenda had her surgery. The article reported on the potential risk of a compartment syndrome in patients who had a Hauser procedure in an attempt to alert orthopedic surgeons to consider this diagnosis in patients having problems in the early postoperative period.

After a pretrial panel reviewed Brenda's case and could not decide unanimously whether there had been a breach of medical standards in her diagnosis and management, McManus asked the judge to set a trial date. Within a month or so, the defense attorney "Harold Bitner," offered a settlement that Brenda and her attorney accepted in lieu of going to trial. What happened before the trial and the settlement turned out to be an unsettling experience for me. Bitner tried something that failed but has bothered me to this day. I had recently resigned from the East Madison Clinic and had accepted a position at the Dean Clinic. This large multispecialty group required a two-year employment period before one could become a partner in the group. This was essentially a probationary period at the end of which they could decide to terminate your employment or make you a partner.

One of the senior and more influential members of the Dean Clinic was an urologist, "Dr. Tony Arthur." One day while I was making my hospital rounds on the floor that had both orthopedic and urology patients, Dr. Arthur approached me as I was reading one of my patient's charts. He said he wanted to talk to me in private.

We walked down the corridor until we came to an empty room and went in. He said he had talked to Harold Bitner, a good friend, who had asked him to tell me that it was a mistake for me to participate as an expert witness against his client. I could not believe what I was hearing and did not want to be any party to this type of intimidation, as subtle as Arthur was trying to make it. I simply told Arthur I felt very strongly that what I was doing was right and did not care what it might cost me personally. As it was, it did cost me the friendship of the surgeon for whom I otherwise had great respect. He refused to acknowledge my presence for many years whenever we crossed paths.

Frankly, I can personally understand the bitterness he had because being the subject of a malpractice suit is a psychologically traumatic experience, which I came to realize in a case involving myself as the defendant. Fortunately, in the years since we have both retired, we have been able to communicate with one another in a civil manner, particularly since we agree on many things both inside and outside of medicine.

As I now reflect on what I consider an attempt to intimidate me to quit as an expert witness, it never occurred to me at the time that I probably had good reason to file a complaint against Bitner with the Ethics Committee of the Wisconsin Board of Attorneys. In retrospect, this probably would have gone nowhere given Bitner's reputation and political influence. I suspect Dr. Arthur would have denied that Bitner had asked him to intervene for him and his client. I learned that success in getting an attorney reprimanded for a breach of ethical standards is difficult to accomplish, as I will detail in a future example.

One of the benefits of my experience in this single case of compartment syndrome was that it animated my interest in the subject. As a result, I eventually decided to do a retrospective study of patients who had been diagnosed with compartment syndrome at both St. Mary's Hospital and Madison General Hospital in the previous ten years. I was able to collect about twenty cases. I determined common threads and, while not finding anything earthshaking, I was able to put together a lecture on the subject. I made presentations at grand rounds at St. Mary's Hospital and at an annual meeting of the Wisconsin Orthopedic Society in Milwaukee. I also used this lecture to teach physician-assistants and residents at the Bugando Hospital in Mwanza, Tanzania, where I worked for a couple of months as a volunteer teacher and surgeon for an organization known as Health Volunteers Overseas.

In addition to the above benefits, I had the good fortune to be on call one weekend when one of the Dean Clinic vascular surgeons asked me to see a patient in the emergency room that had been referred to him from the Watertown Hospital. The patient was a twenty-year-old hockey player, injured in a club game at UW Whitewater. He had sustained a hard blow to his right thigh when he was aggressively checked into the boards. He had been assisted off the ice and gradually developed increasing pain in his thigh. He eventually went to Watertown Hospital, where he was admitted with a suspected vascular injury from bleeding because his thigh had become quite swollen several hours after his injury and X-rays of his femur were normal. He had begun to experience numbness in his thigh and leg. A femoral arteriogram was done, and there was no evidence of damage to the femoral artery or its main branches. He was then transferred to St. Mary's Hospital for further vascular evaluation. Our vascular surgeon saw him first and asked me to evaluate him because he thought the patient must have an orthopedic problem.

When I first saw him, he was lying on a stretcher with his right knee slightly bent, and his right thigh was swollen and tense. Any attempt on my part to bend or straighten his knee was impossible because of the amount of pain it produced to do so. I gathered the necessary equipment to measure the pressures in the muscle compartments of his thigh and confirmed the diagnosis of a compartment syndrome.

His compartment thigh pressure was well over forty millimeters of mercury, so I notified the operating staff that I would be bringing a patient up for a fasciotomy and personally called the anesthesiologist. After his leg was shaved, prepped, and draped, I made an incision, careful not to apply too much pressure on the scalpel.

As the skin, subcutaneous tissue, and fascia were incised, the muscle burst through, causing the scalpel to plunge into it. The appearance of the muscles bursting through the incision was so impressive that I scrubbed out to get my camera and take some photographs that would go along with my preoperative pictures.

He had very little pain postoperatively, except when the saline compresses placed over the wound were changed. After about five to six days, the muscle swelling had gone sufficiently to permit his wound to be completely closed. Serial photographs taken at the time of his post-op visits showed a well-healed incision and eventually a return to a full range of motion in his knee, leaving him no residuals from his condition other than the scar resulting from his limb-saving procedure.

While a thigh compartment syndrome is uncommon compared to compartment syndrome in the leg and forearm, it has been reported. It is often the result of a crushing injury to the muscles that swell from the direct trauma. Another example of how this could happen is if a large weight pinned someone's thigh against the floor or ground. Frankly, this was the first case I had seen, but being aware of the possibility and looking for the criteria made it easy to diagnose.

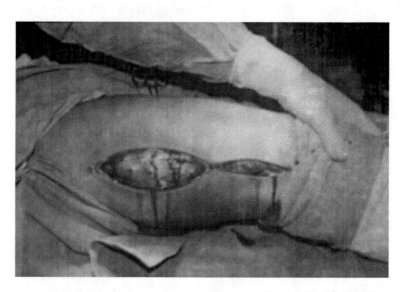

Figure 7 Skin incision made for thigh compartment syndrome

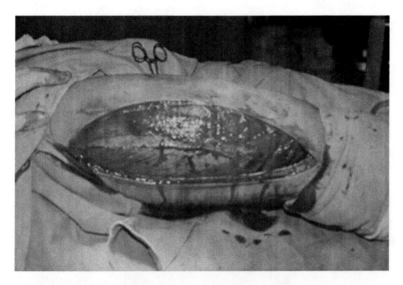

Figure 8 Completed fasciotomy for thigh compartment syndrome

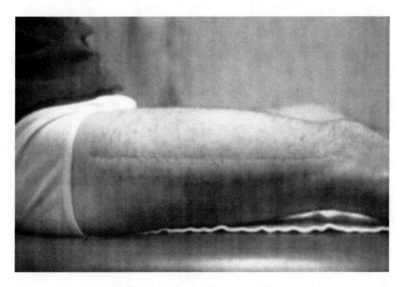

Figure 9 Full knee extension post-op fasciotomy

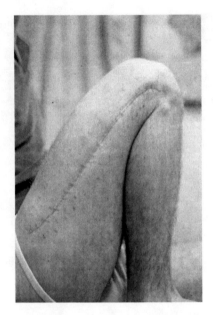

Figure 10 Full knee flexion post-op fasciotomy

I presented this case of a thigh compartment syndrome at a sports medicine conference held at a Wisconsin Orthopedic Society meeting. After giving the history of the case and showing the pre- and postoperative photographs, I was looking forward to hearing the guest speaker, a sports medicine expert from Canada, remark about his experience with the problem. To my surprise and most of the people in the audience, he said he did not think compartment syndrome existed in the thigh. He claimed that what I was treating was something he would have treated with sympathetic nerve blocks in Canada. It was obvious that he had never actually seen a case of this or read the reports others had in their published series.

What he was treating with sympathetic nerve blocks is a condition known as causalgia, where a limb injured from either minor or significant trauma becomes intensely painful because of damage to the peripheral nervous system. There may or may not be swelling, numbness, and painful movement, but at no time is there an increase in the intracompartmental pressures. As it turns out, this "expert" was like a fish out of water in some areas of orthopedic surgery. In Canada, he was an expert in knee ligament and cartilage surgery, giving him a narrow focus, or perhaps because he was near the end of his career he may not have been keeping up with general orthopedics. That is one of the reasons the American Academy of

Orthopedic Surgery publishes the *Orthopedic Update* volumes every few years and the American Board of Orthopedic Surgery requires recertification by examination every ten years of its members.

As it turns out, failure to diagnose a compartment syndrome is one of the leading reasons patients sue orthopedic surgeons for negligence in this country. Given the significant residuals that patients can suffer from a missed or delayed diagnosis, including amputation, this should not come as a surprise.

Lesson 8:
Preparation Is Important if You Are the Defendant in a Malpractice Claim

While my experience in treating most patients in my career will always remain positive, my singular experience with "Delbert Greeley" and his lawyer will forever be a negative one. Mr. Greeley, who held a significant position in the Wisconsin state government, was a patient of Dr. Tim Harrington, a rheumatologist. Mr. Greeley was becoming increasingly handicapped because of osteoarthritis of his knees, and conservative measures no longer benefited him. His arthritis was mostly confined to the inner aspects of both knees. This was in large part because he was bowlegged, and the resultant stress in this type of knee deformity is predominantly on the inner part of the knee, as opposed to the outer side of the knee.

Because he was in his early fifties, which was relatively young for a knee replacement at that time in the history of knee replacements, and because the loss of cartilage was confined to just the one side of the knee, I recommended a tibial osteotomy. The removal of a wedge of bone would change his leg alignment so that there would be more stress on the side of his knee that had relatively normal cartilage and less on the side with little or no cartilage remaining. When this is technically well done on the properly chosen patient, it usually results in a dramatic reduction of pain. The beauty of this procedure, besides the cosmetic and pain relief aspects, is that the surgeon can still do a total knee replacement should the patient eventually wear out the remaining cartilage in his or her knee.

After I explained the procedure, anticipated realistic results and uncommon but possible complications such as infection, nerve, vascular damage, failure to relieve pain, and increased knee stiffness, I recommended that he give this matter serious thought and suggested he should feel free to get a second opinion. Mr. Greeley felt Dr. Harrington's recommendation to see me was sufficient and indicated he wanted to have the procedure on both of his knees done as soon as possible. I indicated to him that he would have to wear a cast for a period of six weeks. I stopped using casts when secure plates and screws became available to immobilize the osteotomy internally several years later. Some cases were done without internal fixation, and immobilization depended solely on a cast extending from the upper thigh to the foot. The patient was allowed to put as much weight on his limb as he could tolerate and usually by six weeks, the osteotomy was healed and the cast removed. On rare occasion, the cast might have to be on for eight weeks, but the determination of healing was always made based on X-ray findings taken at six weeks.

After the cast was removed, the patients work with a physical therapist to regain range of motion of the knee. While many orthopedic surgeons are not willing to admit it, the work that a physical therapist does with our patient plays a major role in the good results we see from our various procedures. I am not saying this because my wife Barbara and daughter Ellen are both physical therapists. Good therapists are not only knowledgeable but are great motivators in setting goals and giving the patient positive feedback. A physical therapist is a crucial part of the team concept of medical care.

When Mr. Greeley came in at six weeks post-op to have his cast removed, he was able to put all of his weight on the operated side and was having significantly less pain than he had prior to his surgery. He was anxious to have the second knee scheduled, which we did at that time, but gave him the next six weeks to regain his range of motion and strength in the muscles. I saw him shortly before the date of his second surgery, and he had made good progress in regaining his strength and knee movement. Three months after the first, I performed his second knee operation, and the length of hospital stay was about the same as his first procedure. The only difference in the hospitalization was changing his cast, because he had a little more bleeding than before. I asked my cast technician, Ken Hanson, who had applied several hundred casts in the past, including experience as a medic in the U.S. Army, to change it. Ken also changed the dressing at the time of the cast change and said the incision looked normal. Greeley made an appointment to return to the clinic approximately ten days after surgery to have a window made in the cast and to have his stitches removed. He decided to spend time after his discharge recuperating at a home he had in Door County, some two hours or so from Madison.

Three days before his scheduled appointment, he began experiencing increasing rather than decreasing pain. Instead of coming to Madison to be evaluated, he decided to stay home. When he came in for his afternoon orthopedic appointment, his cast was windowed, and we found the wound to be infected. I arranged to have him admitted, so he went directly to the hospital from the clinic. I advised him not to eat or drink anything because I was going to take him back to surgery. I was able to take him up to the operating room within a few hours of his admission. I explored his wound and found that the infection had extended down to the bone and had entered the knee. After thoroughly flushing out his wound and knee with a few liters of sterile saline, I installed tubing into the knee and wound that allowed for a continuous instillation of antibiotics into both sites. After taking cultures of the wound, I started him on two powerful antibiotics that covered a broad spectrum of bacteria until we got the results of the cultures. A gram stain (test done to identify organisms) of the infected material showed us that the likely organism was a Staphylococcus. In a gram stain, a drop of pus is smeared onto a clear glass plate, and it is stained with a dye that allows one to identify the category of bacteria present under a microscope. For example, a gram-positive organism might be Staphylococcus or pneumococcus, and a gram negative might be E. coli. The gram stain results are received within an hour of being sent to the lab. The specific nature of the organism and its sensitivity to various antibiotics comes back as a culture report from the laboratory within forty-eight hours.

Fortunately, the organism, which was a Staphylococcus aureus, was sensitive to methicillin, which was one of the drugs I had originally given him. I asked Dr. Kim Hetsko, a specialist in infectious diseases, to see him and give me his opinion on the dosages and length of treatment. Dr. Hetsko approved the dosage and recommended a period of six weeks of antibiotics. We kept him hospitalized for the first two weeks of that treatment to follow his wound closely. When he was discharged, his knee initially was kept relatively quiet in an immobilizing brace. His wound healed well, and, when X-rays showed his osteotomy had healed, we began physical therapy. After six weeks of intravenous antibiotics, there were no signs of any residual infection, not only in the way the leg looked but also based on laboratory tests.

I had told Mr. Greeley that he would likely not get a full range of motion from the second osteotomy because his knee had been immobilized longer than the first knee and because the infection had gained access to his knee. Ordinarily, when someone has a knee joint infection, we try to begin range of motion exercises to minimize adhesions or scarring inside of the knee, which tend to freeze up the joint. He worked in physical therapy for weeks to regain his range of motion but was only able to achieve about 75 percent of the range of motion that he had in his first knee. The physical therapist discharged him after it was felt he had reached maximum benefit from therapy. He returned for his scheduled follow-up appointments with me for the first few months and then stopped coming to the appointments that I had asked him to make.

The next time I heard from Mr. Greeley was through a letter from his attorney. Frankly, I had been expecting that this was what was going to happen when some time after Greeley's last appointment, an attorney from Milwaukee, "Paul Bridges," had requested copies of Mr. Greeley's complete medical record. While I was as disappointed in the result of his second knee range of motion as he was, I was comfortable with the way we managed the infection and post-op care from the initial second surgery. I discussed this with Dr. Hetsko, who agreed that everything done to diagnose and treat him had met the standard of care here or anywhere else. Despite this reassurance, I was destined to have my first encounter with attorneys in a malpractice suit in which I was the person being sued. While I had heard how unsettling this experience is for doctors going through it, I had no idea of the ordeal I was about to be put through.

The first inkling of what was to come happened during my deposition by Attorney Bridges, who seemed to be a pleasant but businesslike man in his early forties. Apparently, to make it convenient for me, the deposition took place in one of the St. Mary's Hospital conference rooms. A court reporter present took notes and taped the deposition. My insurance carrier had chosen the defense attorney with whom I had met previously and discussed the case for at least an hour. His advice to me before the deposition was to answer the questions with yes or no answers and not to enlarge on the answer if possible. He explained that attorneys are taught to go over the deposition with a fine-tooth comb to find any flaws, cracks, or inconsistencies in what was said by the defendant.

After I was asked to identify myself and present my training background and board certification in orthopedic surgery, I was handed a copy of what was supposed to have been the patient's hospital record. I was asked to review it and indicate whether I thought it was a copy of the patient's record. I indicated that it appeared to be the case. One of the first things Bridges then asked me to do was to go to that portion of the chart where the patient's temperature and pulse were recorded so that we could see a graph showing each day divided into four quadrants on the horizontal axis and the temperature and pulse on the vertical axis. Both the temperature and pulse were represented by black lines that went from one reading of the temp and pulse to the next reading, showing four points on the chart for each day. This way one could glance at the graphic and see whether the patient had an elevated temperature and how it varied from day to day.

He pointed out that the temperature line indicated that the patient had a fever while he was in the hospital for his second osteotomy and that on the day he was discharged he still had one. When I saw what he was getting at, I felt angry because I had reviewed the chart several times before the deposition and knew what he was saying was not true. Before going any further with the deposition, I asked that the proceeding be stopped because I wanted to go to the medical records room to retrieve Mr. Greeley's actual chart. I looked at the graphics on the chart in the medical record room and discovered exactly what had been done that gave the false impression that Greeley had a fever during his hospitalization, as well as at the time of discharge.

When nurses chart the graphics at St. Mary's Hospital, they use a red pen to indicate temperature and a blue pen for the pulse. When the chart was copied page for page, everything was printed in black. It was clear to me that Attorney Bridges had been misled by the fact that he could not see colors when in fact he was interpreting the pulse as the temperature. At no time during that hospital stay did the patient have an elevated temperature, as noted in the actual hospital chart. As I walked back to the conference room, I was thinking that clarifying this to Bridges would snip this suit in the bud. When I presented my clarification of his misinterpretation of the record because of the lack of color identifying the proper lines, Bridges was stoic, consulted in a recess with Mr. Greeley, who was also present at the deposition, and returned to ask the remainder of his prepared questions. What I did not know at the time was that he already had two expert witnesses willing to testify against me based only on the information provided to each of them from copies of the chart. When my attorney subsequently deposed his expert witnesses and brought them the clarification of the record, one of his witnesses, an orthopedic surgeon from Milwaukee, withdrew his opinion of negligence. The second expert witness, an orthopedic surgeon from California, said he would still be willing to testify against me. He held no academic position or had any special qualifications other than the fact that a significant part of his income was derived from being a witness for plaintiffs in malpractice suits. Some would call him a professional witness or a "hired gun" while others, like my son Mark, now a medical defense attorney, would refer to him as a "whore."

My attorneys asked who I would recommend to review the records and possibly to testify on my behalf. I recommended three people. The first was a professor in the infectious disease section at University Hospital, Dr. William Scheckler. The second was a professor in the orthopedic surgery department at University Hospital, Dr. James Keene. The third was a respected community orthopedic surgeon, Dr. Eugene Nordby, who had been the chief of staff at Madison General Hospital and one of my mentors when I was a university resident rotating at his hospital. Each of them indicated that there was no evidence of negligence on my part in the management of Mr. Greeley's second osteotomy and in the surgery and care provided by me to diagnose and treat the infection. It should be noted that Bridges deposed our witnesses and that he must have asked probing questions to determine why they came to their conclusion.

The State of Wisconsin required that all malpractice cases, prior to being scheduled for a jury trial, be presented to a three-person panel: an attorney who also presided over the presentations, a Wisconsin-licensed physician, and a layperson. After hearing all the evidence presented to them, the members of the panel were then asked to vote on whether they thought negligence had occurred. The decision of the panel could then be used in a jury trial by either attorney to support the case for the plaintiff or defendant should the suit not be dropped or pretrial settlement made. Despite having the knowledge of what the actual medical record showed and how our experts would testify, Bridges and Greeley decided to proceed with their case against me.

The panel's hearing took place in a downtown Madison hotel conference room that allowed for a set of X-ray view boxes and a long table where the panel sat opposite a chair where the witnesses were seated and questioned by the attorneys. The panel consisted of two men and a woman. One of the men was a family practitioner from Beaver Dam, WI; the other a Madison attorney; and the woman was a schoolteacher from a nearby suburb of Madison.

When Greeley was seated in the witness chair, he attempted to make the point that the second osteotomy was much more painful than the first. He said that when he awoke in the recovery room he remembers asking me why this operation hurt so much. This latter scenario turns out to be a virtual impossibility. I routinely accompanied my patients to the recovery room and waited until the recovery room nurse had recorded the patient's blood pressure, pulse, and respiratory rate. If they were stable, I left the recovery room before the patient was fully awake and able to speak. In addition, patients rarely remembered what went on in the recovery room because of the effects of the general anesthetic and the pain medications they were given intravenously.

Once I left the recovery room, I went to the dictation area to dictate the operative report while it was still fresh in my mind. When that was done, I usually went down to talk to the family, grab a cup of coffee, and wait until my next surgical case is ready. If I was done with surgery for the day, I would see my patients from that day's surgery on the hospital floor or go directly to the office, depending on whether I was running late. It just so happened that day I had another surgery to perform and the average time between cases was about fifteen to twenty minutes.

By the time I completed the next case, Greeley had already been discharged from the recovery room. After I finished seeing my patients in the office, I would usually make post-op rounds at the hospital before going home. Another convincing piece of evidence against the claim made by Greeley was nothing in the recovery room nurse's notes suggested anything out of the ordinary happened. His pain medication requirements in the recovery room as well as during his entire hospital stay for the second surgery were very much like the pain medication requirements in dose and frequency for the first osteotomy.

Of my three witnesses, Drs. Scheckler and Nordby testified in person and were convincing witnesses. Dr. Keene's testimony, which had been videotaped, was similarly persuasive. Bridges's only witness, the orthopedic surgeon from California, had his testimony presented to the panel in written form. I never had an opportunity to see how he tried to circumvent the crux of the case, which was that the temperature record in the patient's actual chart failed to show a fever. I had no idea how Greeley's expert witness was going to show I had been negligent in not making the diagnosis sooner or how the infection could have been treated differently.

When Bridges called me up to testify, he started by asking me to review the X-rays taken in the hospital. I did by first explaining to the panel the nature of the procedure. This showed how it was possible for the infection to extend only a short distance to get into the knee, as happened in Greeley's case. I explained that what they were seeing on the X-ray taken after surgery was the same as the procedure done on his opposite knee.

Bridges tried to make something of the fact that the cast in the hospital was changed by Ken Hansen, our experienced former medic and cast technician, rather than by me. I pointed out that he had probably applied more casts than I had in the last several years. I also indicated that all of the orthopedic surgeons in our five-person department were completely satisfied with his ability to change dressings and apply casts. Whenever there was anything suspicious about the appearance of a wound, he would let us know. I pointed out, as did Dr. Scheckler, that the incubation period of Staph. aureus was from five to ten days. Greeley was discharged on the fifth post-op day, so one would not expect to see any significant findings of an infection in the majority of cases when the cast was changed on the fourth post-op day.

In an almost unbelievable charade, Attorney Bridges went over the graphics of the temperature and pulse from a copy of the patient's chart. He was attempting to justify why we were all spending our time on this case. We had the original chart signed out to us to show the panel exactly what the black lines in the copy represented. After he had completed his questions, the panel had an opportunity to ask me questions of their own. The whole process went from 9:00 AM until about 4:00 PM. As everyone was putting papers away, Attorney Bridges came up to me in an apologetic voice and said, "I just want you to know I was just doing my job." As far as I was concerned, "doing his job" meant not pursuing a case that had no merit. I could do nothing but glare back at him without answering, thereby ending the asinine conversation.

A week later my attorney called to say all the members of the panel had decided there had been no negligence on my part but what he added really upset me. He said that he had talked to the layperson on the panel, who told him that during one of bathroom breaks as she and Attorney Bridges were standing in the lobby, Bridges told her that the hospital had already made a settlement with Greeley. I had no idea why the hospital might have done this if it was true, and it came as a surprise to my attorney and me. I was not even aware that the hospital was being sued. It seemed to me that Bridges's statement was the equivalent of jury tampering and should be considered as unethical or unprofessional conduct.

After receiving this information, I was relieved that the panel voted as they had but was disturbed about the additional information. I decided to write a letter to the Wisconsin State Bar Association, asking their professional conduct committee to review the information about Attorney Bridges talking in private about the case under review with a panel member before she had an opportunity to hear all of the testimony and make a decision.

Almost six months later I received a letter from the Wisconsin State Bar. The letter stated that, after reviewing the information I had provided them and after considerable deliberation, their ethics committee decided there had not been a breach of attorney ethics. I have no idea whether my attorney backed off his claim or the panel member changed her story, but I found it hard to believe that a reprimand of some kind did not result from what allegedly happened.

I was certain that this whole affair with Greeley was going to be put behind me because of the panel decision, but this proved to be wrong. Several months later, I received a letter from an attorney with a law firm in La Crosse, WI, who indicated he was now representing Delbert Greeley. Apparently, Attorney Bridges had advised Greeley he would not be willing to take his case before a jury or Greeley was disappointed in his services and decided to go elsewhere. Whether this was supposed to entice my insurance carrier to make a settlement is pure conjecture on my part, but I never heard from the attorney again and no such settlement was made.

Almost ten years after I last had anything to do professionally with Delbert Greeley, I had an opportunity to read about him in a Madison newspaper in what turned out to be the scandal of 1992. Tim Kelley wrote an article in a recent *Madison Magazine* summarizing it in an ironic way:

> Former Insurance Commissioner [Delbert Greeley], 76, ranked as top poster boy for the "Hall of Shame" tour in 1994, a Democrat road show of unfortunate [Governor] Thompson appointments designed to embarrass the GOP in an election year. [Greeley], who was Assembly speaker in 1963–64, resigned as insurance commissioner in December 1992 and paid a $5,000 penalty to the State Ethics Board in June 1993 for hiring and promoting his roommate to a state job in his office. Should've at least made the guy show up for work, [Delbert].

I would not want anyone to come away from reading this that as an orthopedic surgeon I never made a mistake. Like all physicians, I am human, and to err is human. I have yet to meet a surgeon who has never made an error of judgment or skill during his or her career. Fortunately, in most cases these are minor, and the consequences insignificant. One of the most skillful thoracic, cardiovascular surgeons I have ever met had been sued a number of times. I believe this happened in part because he was willing to take on some of the cases that others might refuse to tackle. Therefore, his complication rate was higher than one less daring. In my private practice career of twenty-nine years, I have been involved in five malpractice cases, including the Delbert Greeley case. None of them went to a jury trial. Three were ruled as no evidence of malpractice. Two were settled out of court for ten thousand dollars because the nature of the error and resulting inconvenience were relatively minor.

The first such case involved fusing the first joint of a male patient's big toe for arthritis that had failed to respond to conservative treatment. The fusion was successful, but I had positioned the toe a few degrees higher than normal for a male but about right for a female, who tends to wear a higher-heeled shoe than a man. Because of this position of the first joint, the toe tended to rub on his shoe, especially when running. I advised him that I would have to revise the position to correct the problem, and he decided to have another surgeon perform the surgery, which worked out well for him. I decided not to contest his claim of negligence as the settlement only involved his time off of work and medical costs, which came to just under ten thousand dollars.

The other case was sheer embarrassment. The patient was a female who had a bone chip in her left ankle that was giving her pain. I recommended that we remove it with an arthroscope through a quarter-inch incision for the scope and the same-sized incision for instruments to extract the bone chip. Unfortunately, the operating room nurse scrub and prepped the right leg and ankle rather than the left while I was out of the room. I had been scrubbing in for the case, and when I entered the room, I did not initially recognize the nurse had prepped the wrong side. I began to perform the arthroscopy on that side. After not finding anything abnormal, we discovered the error, placed a single stitch in the incision over the left ankle, and then scrubbed and prepped the correct side.

The procedure went well from then on, but the patient was upset about having pain in both ankles rather than just one. I elected to admit her to the hospital overnight for observation rather than discharge her the same day, as I would have ordinarily done for this kind of procedure. When the patient decided to sue for the temporary pain, swelling, and the small scar on her normal ankle, I saw no reason not to settle, which again was done for approximately ten thousand dollars. Since that time, the American Academy of Surgery came out with the recommendation that the surgeon's name be written on the limb that is to have surgery, which has eliminated this error when followed. The remaining two cases were determined, as in Greeley's case, not to involve any medical negligence.

It is difficult to get a handle on statistics that show how many times surgeons in America are sued during their careers, but I have heard anywhere from one a year to a handful in an entire career, so my number is probably less than average. At any rate, as a busy orthopedic surgeon I was doing from three hundred to five hundred surgeries per year, which includes innumerable emergency procedures at all hours of the day and night. I feel fortunate with regard to my malpractice history, especially when one considers that this comes from a total of between nine and fifteen thousand surgeries and does not include the management of countless dislocations and fractures that were treated by closed manipulation rather than open surgery. It should be mentioned that physician specialties have different incidences of litigation. Family practice, pediatrics, and internal medicine are on the low end; whereas obstetrics-gynecology, radiology, plastic surgery, neurosurgery, and orthopedic surgery are on the high end. It can even be argued that we have a malpractice crisis in many parts of the country, including New York, Florida, and California. The horrendous settlements that allow some attorneys to become U.S. senators and presidential candidates are responsible for increasing the costs of medical care. Physicians now practice defensive medicine by ordering more lab and X-rays than necessary, even on patients whose diagnosis is in plain view following a good history and physical exam, to avoid a lawsuit.

It is interesting that my son Mark Anton Pellegrino, who graduated from Marquette Law School, should gravitate to medical malpractice defense. I am not certain what made him focus on that area, but he now loves to delve into the medical issues, has become knowledgeable in a number of medical areas, and frequently discusses the cases he is working on with me. One thing that may have influenced him was the fact that I had written a diary of my experience in the Greeley litigation as a form of psychological release. I gave to it to him to read while he was an undergraduate student at Lawrence University. His firm's biggest client, Chicago's Rush University Medical Center, liked his work well enough to offer him a position when one of their top legal staff members decided to leave. He gladly accepted to get out of the rat race of law firms overemphasizing billable hours. This allowed him to have more of a family life, especially on weekends. It is ironic how I found myself in a similar situation in medicine decades earlier.

The final case that I am going to describe is not an orthopedic case. It is an extremely important illustration of the importance of being your own best witness when you have been accused of negligence. This is especially true when the doctor firmly believes that the diagnosis and management of the patient has met the standards of good patient care. The example belongs to a close friend and former associate at the Dean Clinic who specialized in obstetrics and gynecology (ob-gyn). Sadly, it contributed but was not the main reason he decided to retire at age fifty-five.

Unrealistic expectations cause problems in all areas of medicine, and ob-gyn is not an exception. Just like in my case, the doctor's ability to assist his attorney in a malpractice case can and does make the difference between success and failure. This is particularly important when no negligence has taken place. The case is an example of the expectation of a perfect child at birth. When this does not happen, finding fault with anyone who participated in bringing the child into this world is common. It is the number one reason that the cost of malpractice insurance for obstetricians is one of the highest of the surgical specialties. "Dr. James Norseman" followed the young woman throughout her pregnancy, which had been complicated early on by a respiratory infection that did not respond to usual therapy. Consequently, she was referred to an internist, whose recommendations and treatment cleared the infection. Sometime later, she suffered a severe fall that resulted in her being seen on an urgent basis by a musculoskeletal specialist; no serious injury to the mother was found. She subsequently reached her due date without going into labor and ultimately went approximately three weeks over her expected delivery date.

In the period of postdatism, fetal activity determinations were performed weekly and were always normal. On June 27, 1980, she was admitted to the hospital at 10:00 PM with irregular uterine contractions. Through the course of the evening, these contractions did not result in any change of the cervix or descent of the baby's head in the pelvis. Normally, the cervix would start to dilate, and the baby's head would begin to descend lower in the birth canal.

At eight o'clock the following morning, because of continued contractions that were inefficient, the labor was enhanced with the use of carefully monitored intravenous Pitocin, a synthetic hormone that stimulates uterine contractions. According to Dr. Norseman, strict precautions were taken, and a nurse was in constant attendance. The Pitocin was gradually increased, reduced, and again increased on three occasions, but it was not possible to get efficient uterine contractions. During this whole time, the baby was followed on a fetal monitor that gives a tracing that demonstrates the cardiac status of the baby as well as uterine contractions. At no time during the course of labor did the fetus show severe changes on the monitor.

Because they could not get the patient into good labor or to dilate any more than four centimeters, the oxytocin was discontinued, and it was decided to deliver the baby by cesarean section. This was not an emergency cesarean section, and the patient was monitored continuously during the course of the waiting period.

At the time of cesarean section, it was noted that there was meconium, which is the bile-stained contents of the fetal intestine, in the amniotic fluid. In full-term infants, this is seldom found, and when it is, fetal stress is often considered the reason. However, in a post-term delivery, meconium in the amniotic fluid is quite common, even in the absence of stress. While the head was exposed and before the chest of the infant was delivered, a special suction device was used to evacuate the contents of the mouth and trachea so that, when the child took his or her first breath, it would not breathe in the contaminated fluid. The infant was then completely delivered and handed over to a pediatrician, who took over the care and evaluation of the baby from that point on. The infant's Apgar scores were four at one and five minutes. The Apgar score is a measurement of a newborn's response to birth and life outside the womb. Ratings are based on the following factors:

- Appearance (color of pink is good; blue is bad)

- Pulse (pulse over one hundred, good; under one hundred, bad)

- Response to stimulation (none, bad; very responsive, good)

- Activity (or muscle tone where limp is bad; and active movement, good)

- Respiration (absent or weak, bad; crying, good)

Each has a value of zero to two. A high score is ten and the low end is one. A low score alerts a doctor that resuscitation may be necessary, and a high score reassures a doctor that the baby is healthy. Children with cerebral palsy often receive low Apgar scores.

The pediatrician assisted the baby's respiratory efforts by using a mask and inflated bag to assist the infant's respirations along with supplemental oxygen. The child was cared for in the neonatal intensive care unit of the hospital and survived despite a significant mortality rate that can occur with infants born with such a low Apgar score. This infant was eventually diagnosed with cerebral palsy and brain damage.

Five years after the delivery, the family brought a malpractice suit against all of the physicians who had anything to do with the infant's care as well as the hospital. Since Dr. Norseman had been responsible for the mother's care and the delivery of the child, he was one of the main doctors in the suit.

The malpractice suit centered on whether hypoxia (oxygen deprivation) at the child's birth caused her cerebral palsy and brain damage, and, if so, whether Dr. Norseman and the pediatrician had negligently caused those injuries. The plaintiff's attorneys acquired an expert witness who was nationally recognized for his expertise in the interpretation of fetal monitor recordings. This expert indicated that he felt Dr. Norseman had not properly read the fetal monitor tracings that indicated the fetus was under stress.

When Dr. Norseman was put on the witness stand, his attorney asked him about his opinion of the plaintiffs' (baby and mother) expert witness, and he said that he had the greatest respect for his expertise, had read most of what he had written in the medical literature, and used that knowledge in the care of his patients. In fact, Dr. Norseman had read virtually every piece of literature that this expert had published. He found an article published the year before this baby was born in which the expert described the very tracing changes he was now calling abnormal as insignificant changes. It turns out it was not until well after this child had been born that the expert recognized these changes represented fetal stress.

When it came time for Dr. Norseman's attorney to cross-examine the plaintiff's expert, he asked the expert if he recalled the article he had published in December of 1979, approximately six months before the delivery of this child, in which he had described the fetal monitor changes in question as being insignificant. The expert acknowledged that he had published such an article. The attorney then asked, if Dr. Norseman considered him as one of his sources of reliable knowledge in his interpretation of fetal monitor tracings, would he be critical of Dr. Norseman's care and evaluation of this mother and fetus? The expert said that if Dr. Norseman had made his decisions based on the information he had published at the time, he would have nothing to say that was critical of his care of the mother or child. Dr. Norseman simply made it possible for the expert to say that at the time of this child's birth the tracing changes were thought to have no meaning. A few years later, it became evident that they indeed indicated fetal distress. This meant that Dr. Norseman had no reason to treat the patient any differently at that time.

Several other medical experts testified for each side. The experts for the plaintiffs testified that hypoxia caused the baby's injuries, and the pediatrician's ineffective resuscitation was a cause of the hypoxia. The defendants' experts testified that hypoxia did not cause the patient's injuries and that the pediatrician had used an acceptable method of resuscitation. They show that the type of cerebral palsy and brain damage this child showed was typical of a congenital condition and not typical of the type of cerebral palsy and brain damage resulting from oxygen deprivation. They felt that the injury occurred at a much earlier time in intrauterine development and not from oxygen deprivation after the baby's due date or at the time of delivery. The jury absolved Dr. Norseman of any negligence, and while they were critical of the pediatrician for bagging (small rubber bag inflated with oxygen) the baby and not intubating it (putting a tube in the trachea or windpipe), they did not feel this caused any of the baby's injuries.

Had Dr. Norseman not done his research and suggested to his attorney how this should be used in his defense, this case would undoubtedly have had a different outcome.

While no plaintiff or victim suffering from an undesirable result should go unrecompensed when it is unquestionably the result of negligence on the part of a caregiver or hospital, patients should not expect that all such results are their fault. The technological aspects of medical care keep evolving, making it possible to recognize and solve problems sooner. In all fairness, it is critical to evaluate each case on the availability of such knowledge at the time of the alleged incident.

Lesson 9:
Don't Breach the Public Trust—Justice Will Be Served in the End

Madison, Wisconsin, is the state capital and the home of the University of Wisconsin. It has two daily newspapers. One is the *Capital Times,* which many consider a consistently biased and outspoken editorial advocate for the progressive wing of the Democratic Party. The other newspaper, the *Wisconsin State Journal* (*WSJ*), is more moderate philosophically in its editorial slant. Given the liberal nature of Madisonians, the *WSJ* has a distribution that surprisingly far exceeds that of its competitor. One of the columnists for the *WSJ,* "Maureen Dahl," writes columns that vary from public interest to philosophical dialogues, and she may cover national, regional, as well as local issues in her columns. She is an excellent writer, who usually replies personally to individuals who praise or find fault with what she has written.

By way of background, I should note that the three hospitals in Madison had all shared in the care of the trauma patient from the 1950s through the 1980s. By trauma patient, I mean those who were seriously injured in automobile, motorcycle, major industrial, farm, recreational, and home accidents. The development of major trauma centers did not develop until the mid to late 1980s. The national centers of great reputation for trauma training were on the coasts, with one in Baltimore, Maryland, and another in San Diego, California. Maryland's program began in 1968 with helicopters bringing patients into a trauma unit started by world-renowned surgeon Dr. R. Adams Cowley. During this period, the UW Hospital was still located in an antiquated building on University Avenue. Ambulances preferred to bypass UW Hospital because the other hospitals had more accessible emergency rooms and care that was just as good.

The physician leaders in these well-known trauma centers and hospitals with similar prestigious programs formed clinical associations for sharing results in publications and medical meetings around the country. Eventually it was decided that hospitals should be designated as level one, two, or three trauma centers so emergency vehicles carrying patients from accident sites would not only prioritize the injuries but make a decision based on the severity of injury as to what level of hospital to bring the patient. A level one hospital required twenty-four hospital specialists in neurosurgery, orthopedic surgery, general surgery, and vascular surgery, as well as anesthesia. After the University of Wisconsin Hospital moved into their new campus building in 1979, which had space for a helicopter pad, it became the only hospital willing to meet those requirements necessary for the designation of level one trauma center, which it finally received on March 26, 1998.

In the late 1980s, almost two decades before University Hospital had its trauma level designated as level one, columnist Maureen Dahl of the *Wisconsin State Journal* interviewed "Dr. Kenneth Still," a University Hospital neurosurgeon. She apparently chose to do this for an update on patient care at University Hospital. Following this interview, Dahl published a prominent article about Dr. Still and the care of head injury patients at University Hospital titled "UW Hospital ranks high in head injury treatment." After reading the information provided to Dahl by Dr. Still, I felt it was at best inaccurate and mostly self-congratulatory. The article claimed University Hospital neurosurgery department had superior results when compared to two of the major trauma centers in the country. These were centers where residents interested in becoming trauma surgeons, known as traumatologists, were taking their fellowships. University Hospital has not established such a fellowship program as of 2007, despite a level one designation. I saw the article by Dahl as misleading the public and more of a publicity piece than an accurate representation of patient-care comparisons.

I decided to check on the authenticity of the claims made in Maureen Dahl's article. I used the same approach in getting information that I had developed in ferreting out accurate information in the case of Dr. Maurice Mansfield's incompetence. I decided to send a copy of Dahl's column to the chairman of the Department of Neurosurgery of both of the university centers in Richmond, Virginia (Medical College of Virginia), and San Diego, California (University of California). Each department chair then forwarded my letter to the individuals overseeing the studies involving their respective trauma centers. Each of those doctors then sent their chair a reply. These replies were forwarded to me as part of their answer to my letter of inquiry.

Both replies were similar in character. One of the trauma specialists had never heard of Dr. Kenneth Still and indicated that he was not part of any of the national trauma groups that met and reported their work. Dr. Lawrence F. Meyer, associate professor of neurosurgery at the University of California sent me a reply on January 12, 1981: He explained that Dr. Kenneth Still was well-known to him and that this was not the first time that this had occurred. He said that the only long-term answer to Sill's claims was their efforts through the National Traumatic Coma Databank, which included a center at Richmond and San Diego. He pointed out that Dr. Still was most interested in getting into this activity, but his proposal did not meet with the approval of the National Institutes of Health. Meyer thought it was interesting that at the time he submitted his data, the mortality statistics at Wisconsin were certainly no better than those anywhere else in the country.

Once again armed with replies that confirmed my suspicions, I decided to inform columnist Maureen Dahl of the misleading nature of her article. Dahl's response to the copies of the letters from Virginia and California and to my personal comments about that particular column was about as disappointing as the first letter I received from Major General Crouch concerning Dr. Mansfield. Maureen Dahl simply discharged the evidence by saying she did not feel it was her role to get into the middle of a conflict between doctors. I replied to her that this issue was not an argument between doctors but one of journalistic integrity and accurate reporting to the public. She did not reply to this, and I eventually decided to let it go. In retrospect, now some twenty-plus years later, I should have tried going over her head to the editor, but my guess is that there were people at the paper as well as in the university administration who did not want to see the university embarrassed. If that were the case, they would have prevailed in suppressing any criticism.

In June of 2002, the *Wisconsin Regulatory Digest,* a publication of the Wisconsin Medical Examining Board, listed physicians with whom they had issued "disciplinary actions." On that list in 2002 was Kenneth Still, MD, Madison, WI, who was issued a reprimand and had his license limited for one year. The published reasons were as follows: "Provided medico-consulting services with a number of other physicians. The physicians were required to report and share the income with the other physicians, which he did not do. He double-billed some patients which is contrary to Medicaid and Medicare rules." In addition to limiting his license for one year, he was to "provide no fewer than 160 hours of uncompensated community service. He was also required to pay costs of $1,100.00 for their investigation of the complaints."

While I never succeeded in getting any satisfaction from my efforts for what I considered intellectual dishonesty regarding the information provided to columnist Maureen Dahl, I did find it ironic that many years later a more significant dishonesty caught up to Dr. Still. As I have been led to understand, before the University of Wisconsin medical school had an opportunity to discipline him formally, he was allowed to resign from the faculty with a medical disability. I assume this was the result of a very capable attorney.

Lesson 10:
For Doctors Who Become Patients There Are No Guarantee of Success

When it came to good medicine and public interest, Dr. David Noll stood out among his peers. Here was a man of significant physical stature whose demeanor was that of a saint to many who had encountered him over the years. When David was your anesthesiologist, surgeons felt at ease, knowing that their patients were safe. I am certain that every surgeon who worked with David can recall a case or two in which Dr. Noll's wisdom saved the day. One vascular surgeon remembered being in the middle of a case in which blood was being lost. David calmly spoke over the anesthesia screen, which separates the head of the operating table where he was working from the rest of the patient. He told the surgeon, "I think you need to put your finger on it, Doctor, and stop what you are doing until I get this patient's blood pressure restored with this next transfusion." When blood loss is significant, it can be difficult for the anesthesiologist, who is responsible for replacing the lost blood, to keep pace with the loss. David had been there many times and knew when to call for a break to get caught up.

I always wondered why anesthesiologists picked their particular field. Some opine that doctors choose anesthesia because they lack the people skills needed to work with patients for a prolonged period. I suspect that may have indeed been the reason for some anesthesiologists, who even had difficulties with interpersonal relationships with those in the operating room. One such anesthesiologist disliked coming to the hospital in the middle of the night over cases that he saw other surgeons delay until the next day, even if it was not in the best interests of the patient. This particular anesthesiologist would take twice as long to get to the hospital and sometimes three times as long to get the patient set up for the administration of anesthesia while the surgeon waited, knowing full well what the anesthetist was doing to frustrate him.

I suspect the major reason doctors chose anesthesia had more to do with the challenges associated with the specialty. It required a significant amount of dexterity to treat patients successfully with complex techniques to establish an airway with a tube into the trachea in order to deliver different gaseous anesthetics. Other major challenges involved utilizing their knowledge of cardiopulmonary physiology and the effects of the barrage of drugs on heart, lungs, and brain during cases that varied from mundane hernia repair to extremely complex open heart procedures on two- to three-pound neonatal infants to four or five hundred pound, morbidly obese patients.

Dr. David Noll was certainly not one who had any problems establishing relationships with patients or peers. He was chosen to be chief of staff at St. Mary's Hospital, where he set a high standard for physicians like me. He also played a major role in updating the hospital bylaws, not only at St. Mary's but also at Madison General Hospital, where he was highly respected as well. David also gravitated to the more difficult surgical cases, and while surgeons were not allowed to give their preference for anesthesiologist for their cases, patients were able to make such requests. Somehow, those patient requests became a surrogate means for some surgeons to get whomever they wanted at the head of the table.

Despite his busy career, Dr. David Noll enjoyed his time off with his wife and very talented children. They lived on a farm just outside of Madison where his family raised beef cattle that he took great pride in. David's western-style hat was out of place in the doctor's cloakroom in the Midwest, but whenever you saw it there, you knew he was in the hospital.

One morning Dr. Noll entered St. Mary's Hospital emergency room as a patient rather than as an anesthesiologist coming to start his day in the OR. He was in his late fifties and had developed chest pains earlier that morning that concerned him. His wife brought him in. After the emergency physician saw him, a chest X-ray and electrocardiogram were ordered. When David was shown the chest X-ray, which demonstrated a widened mediastinum (the area between the left and right lung that contains the major blood vessels going to and from the heart), he knew he was in serious trouble. A cardiac surgeon, Dr. Michael Shannahan, was called to see him in the emergency room, and after assessing all of the information, he told David that he was going to take him to the operating room. He felt David had a leaking aneurysm of the ascending aorta, which is that part of the main artery that goes from the left ventricle of the heart to the rest of the body. An aneurysm is a bulbous enlargement of a blood vessel that is prone to rupture and cause the patient to lose blood. Aneurysms can be congenital or acquired. Most of those that are acquired result from degeneration of the muscular wall of the artery from atherosclerosis, commonly referred to as hardening of the arteries resulting from cholesterol and calcium deposits.

The operating room was notified and, as luck would have it, one of the two open-heart operating rooms was available. He was typed and cross-matched for blood, and the best operating room crew was made available to take care of this beloved member of the staff. David knew the mortality rate in the procedure to correct the problem he had was extremely high but was glad to be with staff he had so much confidence in. He was aware that of all the hospitals performing cardiac surgery in Madison, St. Mary's Hospital was the busiest and their mortality rate was one of the lowest in the state. He was also aware that the success rate in this particular procedure had a lot to do with the quality of tissues that the surgeon was dealing with, and I am certain he was hoping his body would offer the surgeon the quality that would permit a technical success.

The procedure involves going on cardiac bypass, which allows the surgeon to work on the apex of the heart and major exiting vessels without it beating and eliminates the flow of blood through the site of the surgery temporarily. This permits the accurate placement of stitches and the fabric graft used to replace the ascending aortic aneurysm. The aneurysm itself is removed by cutting above and below it, leaving tissues that are more normal at the remaining ends. The tissues that remain serve as the site to which an appropriate size and length of graft is sewn. Dr. Noll's operation proceeded well until the time of the placement of stitches into the graft. That part of the resected aorta on the end farthest from the heart had reasonably good tissue to place each stitch. On the end next to and including that part of the heart referred to as the annulus, which holds the aortic heart valves, the tissues were of such poor quality that it was like trying to get a stitch to hold in wet tissue paper. Dr. Shannahan meticulously dissected the tissue, trying again to find something that would hold better, but when he finished he knew it was going to be impossible to get the graft to stay in place once the heart pumped blood through it.

A number of key surgical staff and I were in the operating room, silently observing the drama that was taking place. When it became obvious that we were going to lose this wonderful man, there was not a dry eye in the room. I remember the huge sense of loss I felt when my mother succumbed to breast cancer when I was still seventeen years of age. The same feeling returned in that operating room. The legacy Dr. Noll left was enormous. Part of that legacy was his family. For ten or more years his wife, sons, and daughters, including one who was a professional opera singer, sang all the music at the Christmas midnight mass held in the hospital chapel at St. Mary's Hospital. Every year, there was standing room only for that event.

Whereas Dr. Noll was never aware of any disturbance in his aorta, "Dr. William Bailey" had been aware that he had a small aneurysm in his abdominal aorta for a few years. It was small, and the generally accepted treatment for small ones is to observe them with X-rays at regular intervals, since a significant percentage of aneurysms never get any larger than when they are first noticed on a routine abdominal X-ray. The aorta, which carries blood from the heart, begins in the chest or thorax and is known as the thoracic aorta, as it traverses that part of our anatomy. Once the aorta passes through the diaphragm it is called the abdominal aorta, giving off branches or arteries that go to the various organs contained within the abdominal cavity. Just as the thoracic aorta is susceptible to aneurysms, so is the abdominal aorta. In fact, they are significantly more frequent in the abdomen.

Dr. Bailey was a specialist in internal medicine who practiced at both St. Mary's and what is now Meriter Hospital, or the merged Madison General and Methodist Hospitals. Dr. Bailey had to overcome the stigma that sometimes accompanies someone born with a cleft lip and palate and speaks with a mild lisp. He had excellent medical acumen. He was well respected by his peers and especially by the patients he tenderly guided through minor and major medical crises. I was especially endeared to him because he used me as his orthopedic consultant whenever he had a patient at St. Mary's Hospital, where he had only a small percentage of his practice. His partners preferred to admit their patients to Meriter Hospital, since it was so close to their office. It was inconvenient for him to get coverage of his patients from his partners when they had none at St. Mary's Hospital.

Early one evening, Dr. Bailey experienced spontaneous, severe abdominal and back pain and was brought to Meriter Hospital emergency room. He actually told the emergency room physician that he had an abdominal aortic aneurysm and thought that it was now leaking. Being aware that one has an abdominal aortic aneurysm is not a particularly unusual occurrence, as they can usually be clearly seen on routine abdominal X-ray due to their calcified margins. An aneurysm that is no larger than three centimeters is simply followed by the patient's physician annually, and if it gets progressively larger, it is removed or bypassed with a graft. A significant percentage stay the same, so that regular follow-up evaluations avoid unnecessary surgery.

Dr. Bailey asked to have the vascular surgeon on call come in to evaluate him, but, when the vascular surgeon was called by the ER doctor, he was told that he would not come in until they got the results of a computerized tomography (CT) scan. Getting a CT scan necessitates getting a radiologist to read it and communicate with the ER doctor and/or vascular surgeon. This all takes valuable time, so that by the time the CT scan was done, proving Dr. Bailey to be right in his own diagnosis, which was that his aneurysm was not only leaking but was extending its way up the aorta, damaging some of its tributaries supplying blood to his various organs. At least an hour or more had elapsed from when Dr. Bailey entered the ER to the time Dr. Bailey had gotten to the operating room.

The procedure to remove the aneurysm and replace it with a graft went well, but the vascular surgeon may not have appreciated any damage done to the tributaries that fed blood to his bowels. Dr. Bailey survived the initial procedure but had a stormy postoperative period. Within a couple of days, it became apparent that his abdomen was becoming distended and his bowels were not functioning. Because of increasing abdominal pain and signs of toxicity, he was taken back to the operating room, where the surgeon discovered he had gangrene of a large section of his bowel that had to be removed. By this time, his kidneys, which were also fed by tributaries from the abdominal aorta, began to fail, and in a few days, he expired from the complications that, at least in part, may have resulted from a delay in getting him to the operating room during a critical time.

Surgeons often use the term *golden period* to refer to the ideal time interval from the onset of symptoms to the time those symptoms are treated. When that time interval is exceeded, the results can vary from fair to disastrous, as I believe probably happened in this case.

Lesson 11:
Medical Fiefdoms Exist That Are Power- and Income-driven

As in all fields of endeavor, competition is usually a good thing. We see it in the automobile industry when one manufacturer develops a popular model, as Ford did years ago when it built the Mustang. Those first Mustangs were relatively economical and stylish, so much so that other manufacturers eventually designed similar cars to keep up with the standard set by Ford. Of course, companies like Ford also spent millions of dollars on advertisements to enhance their image in the marketplace, something that had been avoided for decades in the medical profession. I think this was probably because self-advertising was not thought to be in the best interest of the patient. However, extensive advertising and marketing continue to be common practice in the legal profession. I suppose the ethics of treating the contents of ambulances rather than chasing ambulances might account for one of the reasons the medical profession was slow to get involved in these practices.

Now that we have crossed the bridge into the twenty-first century, those prohibitions have for the most part disappeared. We now see slick advertisements by plastic surgeons, orthopedic surgeons, cardiologists, and on and on. Hospitals trumpet their various departments on billboards, television ads, and the newspapers. Almost simultaneous with this new medical showmanship, the drug manufacturers began to advertise directly to the consumer, bombshelling them with all sorts of drugs to cure problems such as erectile dysfunction, hypertension, high cholesterol, baldness, and so on.

During the first half of my career as a physician, the main way to compete for patients was to provide the kind of care and results patients expected. Satisfied patients invariably would tell their friends and relatives about you, and this resulted in new patients. At the same time, if a physician was a specialist, it was critical to develop good working relationships with primary care physicians who were in internal medicine and general practice. It was not only important to provide excellent care to a referring doctor's patients but to also communicate with that doctor so that he or she was aware of the patient's progress and could answer questions family members might ask. Failure to do so might result in the loss of doctor referrals.

Patients in rural communities may have only one local option for a family physician. Most of the doctors in those communities were well liked and trusted. They often worked long hours, took few vacations, and provided care for more than one generation of a given family. Many of them preferred to have patients requiring hospitalizations admitted to their local hospital, which might only have fifty beds, rather than travel to the "big" city for their care. Some of these small-town doctors constantly pestered specialists to come to their rural hospitals to perform procedures. The orthopedic department of the Dean Clinic, which I had recently joined after practicing for five years at the East Madison Clinic, had agreed to send one of its members to a hospital in Sauk City to perform minor procedures, such as ganglion cyst removal and carpal tunnel nerve releases. Both of these procedures could be done under a local or regional anesthetic. Since these patients would not require an overnight stay under ordinary circumstances, it would not present a logistical problem of returning in the middle of the night from thirty or more miles away to take care of any complications that might occur with hospitalized patients.

One uncomfortable situation convinced me that even minor procedures put us at risk. Only nurse anesthetists without the supervision of an anesthesiologist served the hospital operating rooms in Sauk City, WI. A male patient had been referred to me for removal of a benign growth on his lower left leg. I was to perform his procedure while he was under a regional anesthetic, which involves using a tourniquet on the leg several inches or more above the tumor to control bleeding and confine the anesthetic to the area below the tourniquet. The blood is removed from the leg by tightly wrapping it with an elastic bandage and then a blood pressure tourniquet is used to prevent the return of blood to the leg. A needle is threaded into a vein along with a tiny catheter below the tourniquet before the blood is removed from the leg. Once the blood has been removed, the tourniquet is elevated, and a specific volume of anesthetic, known as lidocaine, is injected into the patient's leg. This fills the collapsed blood vessels and goes to the tissues where the surgery is to be performed.

Ordinarily the tourniquet is elevated for between twenty and sixty minutes, during which time the lidocaine becomes physically bonded to the tissues, resulting in very little of it escaping into the general circulation. The limb is usually scrubbed with soap and an antiseptic is applied to the skin before the surgery is performed; this takes several minutes, giving the anesthetic a chance to numb the tissues.

The surgical prep never took place. Several seconds after the nurse anesthetist injected the lidocaine, my patient became extremely apprehensive, sat up, and started convulsing. Fortunately, we had an anticonvulsant medication available in the operating room, and within the next ten minutes, he was back to normal except for a headache. As it turned out, the anesthetist had essentially given him a large dose of lidocaine that had gone directly into the patient's circulation because he had not elevated the pressure on the tourniquet sufficiently high enough to prevent this. The anesthetist was reportedly experienced in this technique and had done it a number of times successfully in the past.

I elected to abandon the procedure rather than risk any further problems. After we took the patient to the recovery room to continue to monitor his vital signs, I went to the waiting room to tell his wife what had happened. She was shocked at the potential harm that might have come to her husband. I had an uncomfortable feeling that something was going to come of this from a medical-legal standpoint based on her reaction. After speaking with her, I placed a call to the family doctor who had referred the patient and had desired the work to be done locally. I told him of my concerns about the patient's wife and asked that he spend some time reassuring her that this was not my fault, although most attorneys would try to implicate me. He must have done a good job, as I never heard about the case again. I continued to be uneasy about working in that environment and was pleased when one of the orthopedic residents decided to set up practice there the next year after she completed her training at the university.

While this episode concerning my experience at the Sauk Hospital was a digression from the patient-possessive doctors, it was just one such doctor on that staff who illustrates the purpose of this lesson of the book. His name was "Dr. Boris Guteranz," and his office was in the town of "Complex," WI. Dr. Guteranz was born in one of the Baltic countries and had many memories of his experiences living there as a youth when the Nazis took over his country. One of his memories remains vivid in my mind. He recalled it for a number of us one day in the doctors' surgical lounge at St. Mary's Hospital. He told us about the time he saw, apparently within relatively close range, the Nazis surround a synagogue where most of the Jews in their small town had gone to seek shelter. The Nazis placed gasoline around the wood structure and burned it to the ground with all the people inside. He recalled the screams from those inside and the smell of burning human flesh that persisted in the area for days on end.

Dr. Guteranz frequently arranged for a Dean Clinic surgeon to perform surgeries for one or more of his patients so that he could be there to assist in the surgery, collect an assistant's fee, and ostensibly demonstrate his concern for his patients. Local family doctors in Madison occasionally asked to assist a surgeon, even though they knew that St. Mary's Hospital was one of the training hospitals for the university residents. As a result, there was usually a resident available to assist and learn in gynecologic, urologic, general surgery, and orthopedic cases. Other doctors from outlying communities did not want to spend time away from their practices to assist surgery in Madison. Dr. Guteranz let it be known to all his patients that he preferred that they did not see any other doctor or specialist without first consulting him. I do not know whether he did this with his patients' best interests in mind or his own. A number of folks from Complex had friends from neighboring areas who were very happy with a specialist who had treated them and recommended that specialist to their friends if they had similar problems. Patient referrals are commonplace in every doctor's practice, and that is how practices grow. In Dr. Guteranz's case, however, if one of his patients decided to see someone without his recommendation and he learned of it, he dropped them. That seems to be a high price to pay for exercising one's right to freedom of choice and represents a classic example of a patient-possessive doctor.

Primary care physicians are not the only patient-possessive doctors. Surgeons who have been in practice for a decade or more were not infrequently offended when they perceived that a younger partner was trying to "steal" a patient. I recall one specific incident that occurred in the hallway of the surgical suites at one of the Madison hospitals. A senior surgeon approached his younger partner and asked why he had operated on one of his former patients, after the younger doctor had been consulted first on his on-call day. Each department with more than one member worked out a schedule of on-call days so that they could get home at more reasonable hours when not on call. The responsibilities of the on-call surgeon are to take care of emergency cases, see all consults requested of the surgery department, and answer calls from nurses or patients. Apparently, the surgery had been an elective procedure, and the patient had had a number of procedures performed by the senior surgeon in the past several years. The younger surgeon stood his ground. As they stood face to face with several of the staff in observance, the senior surgeon thumped his index finger on the chest of the younger surgeon and said, "This is not the way we do things around here, Doctor." Fortunately, calmer voices prevailed, and the situation was defused. But I do not think the two of them spoke to each other for a number of months.

I must say that I have always felt patient loyalty was something a doctor earned. I found that most of my patients were indeed loyal. I do not know whether the senior surgeon's former patient had inquired about his availability, and, if so, whether the younger surgeon replied positively or negatively. I will say one thing in that regard: whenever I had a patient who desired a second opinion, I was never offended. In fact, I would be quite happy with that request. If, however, the patient decided to have surgery done by the doctor who gave them the second opinion and then came back to see me because they were not happy with the results, I usually referred them back to the original surgeon. The exception was when the surgeon personally asked me to take care of his problem. That rarely happened. I felt directly responsible for patients who were loyal to me but saw no obligation to be responsible for patients who sought their care elsewhere after first being evaluated by me. One such case cost me the friendship of a cardiologist's wife, a lovely woman, admired by many for her varied talents. Her husband subsequently told me he completely understood my reasons and had no problems with my decision.

His wife's mother was a delightful, slightly vain woman who had previously seen at least two orthopedic surgeons in Milwaukee whom I knew to be excellent orthopedic surgeons. She had degenerative arthritis of her knee, which had been treated with anti-inflammatory medications and cortisone shots. After they had discussed surgical procedures with her, she asked her son-in-law what she should do, and he recommended she see me for my opinion. After my evaluation of her knee and X-rays, I told her that she would benefit from a total knee replacement and that the degeneration had progressed to the point where any lesser procedure would either not be successful or would only be temporarily and partially successful.

After talking with her, I realized that her expectations were greater than what the procedure might be expected to achieve, including a joint replacement. Getting a new knee with surgical implants is not the same as restoring the knee that you had when you were twenty years old. I also was not convinced that she was aware of the magnitude of the commitment to the rehabilitation process required of total knee patients. I told her exactly what I would tell all my patients with her problem. When she reached the point that she could no longer live with the pain and disability, she should seriously consider having a knee replacement. I assumed that since I was seeing her as a second opinion she would go back to Milwaukee and have one of the surgeons she had seen there perform the procedure. Although I did not tell her this, I would have been willing to do her surgery at that time if she had insisted.

Unbeknownst to me, she traveled to Flint, Michigan, where she saw another orthopedic surgeon with a national reputation in arthroscopic surgery of the knee. He performed arthroscopic debridement of her knee and a proximal tibial osteotomy. These procedures involve looking in the knee with an instrument about the diameter of a pencil and, through small incisions, inserting hand and power instruments to remove frayed, torn, or loose pieces of cartilage or bone and bone spurs. The proximal tibial osteotomy involves taking a wedge of bone out of the upper end of the tibia, closing that gap, and securing the bones with a small plate and several screws as previously described. The former procedure removes some of the irritants inside of the knee and the latter procedure realigns the weight bearing to the side of the knee with lesser involvement, similar to the effect you get from rotating your automobile tires.

Unfortunately a year after the procedures in Flint, Michigan, she was having the same symptoms that she had before the surgery. That did not surprise me. When she came back to see me, I reexamined her, reviewed her X-rays, and listened to her complaints. I told her that she had reached the point where she should have a knee replacement. I also told her I was not comfortable with accepting her as my patient and reassured her that the surgeons in Milwaukee would be able to do an excellent job for her. Unfortunately, this did not sit well with the patient or her daughter, who had not accompanied her to my office on any of her visits. I have had my share of patients with unrealistic expectations, and it can be psychologically burdensome to care for them, particularly if there are any complications.

Lesson 12:
Doctors Who Do Not Quit Soon Enough May Cause a Medical Tragedy

"Dr. Samuel First" was one of several physicians, including the Dean brothers, James and Joseph, who started the Dean Clinic that subsequently became the Dean Medical Center, with over three hundred providers and a couple of thousand employees working in Madison and the surrounding communities. Dr. First specialized in obstetrics and gynecology. When he started his practice in Madison, he was one of the few specialists in this field. During his years in practice, he delivered several thousand babies, including my loving wife, Barbara. He was asked to stop operating at nearly seventy years of age.

As it turned out, one of the major reasons was how he had mismanaged the care of my wife's mother, Dorothy Werth. Dorothy, who had given birth to four children, developed stress incontinence, which results from a stretching of the tissues extending from the bladder to the urethra, leading to the involuntary loss of urine when coughing or sneezing. Many women who have delivered one or more children develop this problem. Dorothy was in her fifties when she approached Dr. First about the problem and mentioned that she also had occasional spotting of blood coming from the vaginal area. He told her it would be smart to take care of both problems at the same time and recommended a vaginal hysterectomy and repair. The hysterectomy involves the removal of the uterus, either through the vagina or through an abdominal incision. The repair portion of the procedure involves tightening the soft tissues that have been stretched, thereby taking care of the incontinence problem.

When Dr. First performed the procedure, he neglected to do curettage of the uterus before removing it. Curettage, known as a D & C, involves dilating the uterine opening and inserting a curet that is used to scrape the lining of the uterus for an immediate biopsy report called a frozen section. A frozen section is done by rapidly freezing a tissue specimen, cutting an extremely thin slice of it, staining it with dyes, and looking at it under a microscope. This tells the surgeon before he removes the uterus whether the cause of the spotting was from a benign or malignant process. It is important to know that before removing the uterus, because, if the tissue obtained from the scraping indicates that there is cancer, then the uterus is not removed until after the patient has undergone radiation treatment. Statistically, this has been shown to reduce the incidence of the cancer spreading and therefore significantly improves survival. If this is not done at the time of the surgery, then the patient is subjected to external beam radiation within a couple of weeks of the hysterectomy.

To his embarrassment, the report from the pathologist, which came two days after Dr. First had removed the uterus, showed that there was indeed cancer in the uterus. It was then necessary for her to go through several weeks of radiation therapy while her surgical repair was still healing. The effect of radiation is to kill cancer cells that are rapidly replicating. Unfortunately, the cells important to repairs are also damaged, which condemned the repair for incontinence to failure. While she was a survivor from the uterine cancer, she did have to undergo another repair by one of Dr. First's younger associates; Dr. Norseman. As I understand it, Dr. First was in his mid-to-late seventies at the time of Dorothy's surgery. It was the last case he ever took to the operating room before it was suggested he retire by the clinic administration and his partners.

The second physician who should have quit doing surgery was one of the few remaining general practitioners at St. Mary's Hospital who was still doing surgery in the hospital operating room. He had been in practice for almost forty years and had scheduled a vein stripping on one of his longtime patients for varicose veins. Varicose veins represent a condition that results from the one-way valves in the veins becoming incompetent, thereby allowing dilatation of veins prominently seen through the skin of the legs; this is frequently associated with lower leg or ankle swelling, and leg fatigue. The patient was a woman he had seen since her youth, and he had delivered all of her children. There was a significant bond between this patient and her doctor because he not only delivered her children but also made house calls and treated all of her children's numerous illnesses and injuries. This is seldom seen now because of the changes made in the care of patients. "Hospitalists" now usually take care of hospitalized patients, and primary care doctors primarily do office practices in many areas of this country.

A vein stripping can involve removal of just a few veins, or it can involve removal of most of the superficial venous system. The deep system of veins and their valves are less often affected because leg muscle contractions contribute to the venous return of blood to the main vessel in the pelvis and abdomen known as the vena cava, that in turn returns the blood to the heart. Part of the procedure requires putting a ligature (or tie) around the main superficial vein in the groin area and cutting between two ligatures before stripping out the system of veins below this large vein. Unfortunately for the patient, her elderly doctor mistook the femoral artery that provides the major blood supply to her lower extremity for the large superficial vein in that area. As a result, the patient's leg was without an arterial blood supply for some time before it was recognized. The patient ended up requiring an amputation some time later.

The family doctor was overwhelmed with guilt and could not get up the courage to see his patient as she was recovering from her amputation. Despite his obvious mistake and tragic consequence, his loyal patient was unwilling to initiate a malpractice suit against her doctor. Her family insisted that she consult with an attorney, and she finally reluctantly agreed to do so. The attorney she saw was John Moore, someone I knew well and would see often in Madison ice arenas, as our children played youth hockey together. John told me that the thing that bothered his client more than losing her leg was that her doctor never came to see her in the hospital while she was recovering from her amputation. While I do not pretend to know that much about psychiatry, her doctor must have been devastated by his mistake. I believe he just could not face her after letting her down when she had placed so much trust in him. Patients of that generation venerated their doctors, sometimes to a fault, and were not afraid to express those strong emotions, not only in words but in deeds as well. Some of my most loyal patients would knit things or bake cookies, cakes, and homemade fudge to bring to me at Christmas time. I am certain that he had dozens of patients who did the same. If we start to believe all the praise that is heaped upon us by our grateful patients, we can sometimes get an unrealistic sense of infallibility.

Being able to process this type of high praise is important for physicians. If a physician is unable to do so, it can account for the difference between the doctor who practices with humility and the one who practices with vanity. Unfortunately, some of desired characteristics in students now being admitted to medical schools tend to be directed to the latter character trait, interpreted as confidence, rather than humility.

I can remember a perfect example of that during my years as a medical student. In my class of 1964 at UW medical school, there were only three women admitted in just under one hundred students. Near the completion of our second year of medical school, one of the three women was dropped from the class because one influential male member of the faculty decreed she just did not have a "forceful enough personality" to make a good physician. She was admittedly rather shy but was as bright as anyone in the middle third of our class. There is no question in my mind that she would have made a wonderful pediatrician or family practitioner. Most of us knew the decision to drop her from our class was a travesty. Because of our own interests in self-preservation, none of us banded together to object to this improper action for fear of what it might do to our own standing in our class. I cannot imagine that someone like this pompous professor who tried to do this now would not face a lawsuit for doing so.

Lesson 13:
Orthopedic Doctors Create New Joints and Lifetime Memories

While serving in the Air Force, a young woman, Joy White, in her twenties with two young children, came into my office complaining of pain in her leg. She was the wife of an Air Force sergeant. She was originally from Tennessee and spoke with a soft Southern accent that was pleasing to the ear. She had a history of leg pain of several months' duration, which was not associated with any injury. It was getting progressively worse. She pointed to her shin as the area of her pain. There was no evidence of swelling, discoloration, or increased temperature over this area. When I put digital pressure on the front of her tibia about a third of the way down from her knee, she complained that it hurt for me to do this. When she walked, she seemed to favor that side, but only slightly.

I obtained an X-ray that showed a patchy area of decreased bone density. Bone density on a plain X-ray is represented by the degree of whiteness of the bone. The outside of a bone is usually very white or dense; whereas the center of the bone is less dense or white. Most of her decreased bone density, which involved her tibia, was in the center, but the outside was slightly involved as well. There were two main considerations for her diagnosis. One was a low-grade bone infection, and the other possibility was a tumor of some kind. There were other possibilities, but they were significantly less likely. After telling her what we found, I recommended that we explore this area. I told her if it was an infection I would open a window in her bone to drain out any pus and we would place her on antibiotics. I told her that if it was a tumor we would do what we thought best, but if it required an amputation I would talk to her about the type of malignancy and how it would best be treated before proceeding.

At the time of her surgery, after I had teased the muscles off with an instrument known as a periosteal elevator, the external surface of the bone looked normal. Using her X-rays, I judged how far from her knee the problem area was located. I made a small window in the bone and lifted off a small section of the bone in that area. A window is made by using a drill to make four or more holes in the bone at the corners of the window and then cutting the bone with a power or hand tool to create a piece of bone that can be lifted away from the rest of the bone. Beneath this window, the bone did not appear normal. There was gray tissue about the consistency of raw liver that occupied this space. I removed a small specimen and sent it to the laboratory. We waited for the report before proceeding. The pathologist reported that the tissue was very cellular and that he saw a rare mitosis (cell nucleus dividing into two). He was not certain what this was going to be until he had done the permanent sections.

Since he had not come out and said this was definitely malignant I decided to make a much larger window and remove all of the tissue with an instrument that looks like a soupspoon with sharp edges connected to a handle about the size of a golf club shaft. The tool, called a bone curet, comes in many sizes. After curetting out all of the bone that appeared abnormal, I took bone graft from one side of her pelvis and filled the void. I had decided to do this to save her another possible operation if this turned out to be a benign process.

Most others would have simply closed the wound after the biopsy and waited to see what the permanent biopsy report showed. The latter process is the preferred method and the way I had been taught, but sometimes it is necessary to make an exception. The permanent biopsy report came back two days later, and the diagnosis of an adamantinoma was made. This turns out to be one of the lowest-grade malignancies that occur in bone; it grows slowly and does not spread to other areas until it is far advanced.

I discussed the diagnosis with the patient and my impression that I had removed the entire tumor that was exposed to the naked eye. We both decided to see how this healed and to follow up with X-rays at scheduled intervals. I was able to follow her for little over a year, and her X-rays showed that the bone graft healed very nicely and had replaced the patchy area of her original X-rays with what looked like normal bone. She had become free of all the pain she had prior to her surgery, so it appeared to me that we had dodged a bullet by doing it the way I had rather than doing an amputation or some other form of treatment. Joy was very happy with her result and grateful to me for all that I had done for her.

After I left the service, I would get Christmas cards from her for the first several years. About ten years after her surgery, I got a call from her. She told me that she had started having some pain again and that she had gone to the Campbell Clinic in Memphis, Tennessee. She was told that her adamantinoma had recurred, and they were advising an amputation of her leg. She insisted that I do the surgery. I asked her to arrange to have her X-rays sent to me at the Dean

Clinic and that I would call her back. The X-rays showed that the tumor had recurred very close to the original site and, in fact, did not look as bad as the original in terms of size of patchy decrease in bone density. I agreed to perform her surgery after I had a chance to examine her in my office.

Joy came up to Wisconsin. A number of bone cancer centers had been reporting success with limb salvage procedures for certain malignant bone tumors; the process involved removing the entire bone in some cases and replacing it with a cadaver bone or metallic replica of all or part of the bone. After examining her and again reviewing her X-rays, I told Joy that I thought I could save her limb by performing a limb salvage operation in which I would remove the majority of her tibia and replace it with the fibula from her opposite leg.

The removal of a large segment of the fibula from a leg was a procedure I had done for compartment syndrome of the leg in order to decompress all four compartments of the leg. This was a technique developed by Dr. Thomas Whitesides of Emory University in Atlanta, Georgia. The beauty of this technique is that one leaves enough of the upper and lower ends of the fibula so those parts that remain still function normally at the knee and ankle. The fibula itself is not a weight-bearing bone; whereas the tibia is. Patients who have had this procedure, referred to as a fibulectomy, can bear full weight on that side soon after the procedure.

Joy was ecstatic that I was not going to amputate her leg and had complete confidence in what I had recommended. At the time of surgery, I removed her tibia from about two and one half inches below her knee to about three inches above her ankle. I took with the bone a thin layer of the muscles surrounding the bone. I measured the length of the tibia I had removed and removed the fibula from her opposite leg, taking a segment about an inch longer than the removed tibia. This allowed me to place the fibula into the medullary canal of both the upper and lower end of the tibia, which is known as skewering. The leg with the tumor removed was placed in a cast that I bivalved (split each side with a cast-saw) in order to get at access to her incision and allow for swelling to occur. I only put a dressing and elastic bandage on the bone donor leg. The next day, we got her up in a wheelchair, and a few days later we started physical therapy, where she used crutches and began bearing full weight on her donor leg.

At the time of discharge from the hospital, she had almost no pain in her donor leg and was bearing full weight on it. Both of her leg wounds healed and her sutures were removed before she went home with a new cast. I did not allow any weight on her casted leg for several weeks. When it looked like the graft was growing to the two remaining parts of her tibia, I started her with only a slight amount of weight on it. It became apparent after about six months that, while the lower end had bonded nicely, the upper end of the graft had not bonded with the tibia. This meant I was going to have to freshen up that end of the tibia and fibula and add some additional bone graft, which I took from her pelvis. In addition, I placed a screw across the fibula and into the tibia to give additional stability. By securely fixing her intact fibula to the upper tibia nonunion site, the stress was reduced on the area that failed to heal. This functioned like an internal splint. This procedure worked, and the upper end of the fibular graft bonded to her tibia within a couple of months.

What normally happens over a period of time when the fibula is used to substitute for the tibia is that the fibula gets bigger and eventually remodels itself so that after a number of years it looks exactly like a normal tibia. It is important not to allow the patient full weight bearing too soon, as the undersized bone may fracture during this remodeling process. This commonly presents itself as a stress fracture, which is seen as a hairline, almost undetectable, break. This occurred a time or two with Joy, but only meant she had to go back on crutches for a few weeks until her pain disappeared. To reduce the number of trips she made to Wisconsin from Tennessee, she was able to make connections with an orthopedic surgeon who was willing to see her and obtain X-rays that he would mail to me. It has been well over twenty years since I did that limb salvage procedure. Joy is now happily married for the third time and enjoying her grandchildren.

During our trips to Florida, my wife and I have stopped in the Nashville, Tennessee, area a couple of times to join Joy and her husband for dinner at a local restaurant. Hugs and kisses are always exchanged, and my wife understands.

On January 26, 2007, *Newsweek* magazine published an article written by Sarah Childress titled "Healing the Wounded," which described how the "military had rewritten the book on wartime surgery to combat the wave of injuries in Iraq and Afghanistan with innovative strategies for helping fallen warriors." Those innovations had to do with controlling bleeding with coagulant powders combined with direct wound pressure in extremity injuries and a special vacuum pump used to remove dead tissue from wounds, permitting earlier wound closure, which substantially reduced wound infections. I loved this article because it showed that necessity is the mother of invention, especially when it comes to the surgical fields. I developed one of my own "inventions" but for different reasons during my first several years in practice.

At times in orthopedic surgery, it is necessary to have an assistant hold a leg, especially during a procedure that involves working on the entire circumference of a limb. This can be a fatiguing job and may eventually bother one's back if the limb is heavy. Having had my share of back problems, I decided that a unique way to remedy this would be to suspend the leg in the air using a sterile pin through the heel, which was connected to a traction bow that in turn was connected to a sterilized aluminum chain. I would then pass a hook through one of the links at the appropriate length. This whole apparatus was connected to the ceiling by a sterile metal rod that passed through a plate I had installed in the ceiling of one of the orthopedic operating rooms. The sterile rod had a hook on each end so that it could be hooked into the plate as well as through one of the chain links. Instead of using a pin through the heel, I often used sterile cotton webbing and wrapped it around the ankle or wrist as a stirrup to suspend the limb using the sterile chain and rod as already mentioned.

In one memorable case, this apparatus turned out to be particularly useful. A ten-year-old boy, while doing farm chores at 5:00 AM, got his leg caught in a silage auger used to convey silage out of a silo into an area where the cows feed. Once caught, the auger proceeded to amputate his foot, clean all of the muscles off his leg below the knee, remove all of the skin from his leg up to his groin, and cake the muscles of his thigh with thick silage. I knew if I did not remove the dead and contaminated tissue and all of the silage and convert it to a surgical wound he would undoubtedly die of gas gangrene from a bacterial infection. I put a pin through the end of his tibia, suspended the leg at a forty-five-degree angle, and initially "Waterpiked" it with several liters of sterile saline. I then physically scraped every bit of foreign body from the muscles encasing his femur with a scalpel and irrigated it with the pulsating jet stream of saline again until I was convinced that it was thoroughly clean. I then removed the bone not covered by muscle, which included his tibia, and knee.

My plastic surgery associates were amazed how clean the wound looked when we took him back to the operating room several days later for the first of his skin grafting procedures that eventually covered his entire thigh. They used a mesher to allow the skin graft to be expanded because there was such a large area to cover and they wanted to limit the amount of donor graft they would have to take. The mesher creates a myriad number of tiny slits in the skin so that it can be stretched to cover tissue up to 40 percent more than unmeshed skin. Meshed skin graft initially looks like you placed a screen with larger than normal openings over the part you are grafting. The open areas within this net of skin rapidly fill in with skin by growth from the filaments of skin around the voids. The patient was eventually fitted for an above-knee prosthesis, which was a lot better than a funeral.

While working at the East Madison Clinic, I was asked to see an eight-year-old girl who was had begun to limp because of pain in her knee. She had not had any recent injury or other medical problems. Her mother accompanied her, and I examined her, with the only positive finding being tenderness in the end of her femur adjacent to her kneecap. I obtained an X-ray that showed changes consistent with a malignant bone tumor called osteogenic sarcoma, which is the same tumor that resulted in Edward Kennedy Jr. losing his leg in 1973 at twelve years of age. I confirmed the diagnosis with the radiologist and then advised the patient's mother that I thought an amputation would be the only thing that would save her daughter's life, as radiation and chemotherapy were not effective at that time with this particular malignancy.

I had done a great number of amputations in the lower extremity, but this was the first time I was faced with doing it on a child, which gave me great pause. I will never forget the look on this girl's face when she came back from the operating room and saw that I had removed her leg at the upper thigh. I cannot remember her smiling anytime during that hospitalization. Her incision healed very well, and I placed the stump of the amputation into an elastic stocking that was designed to eliminate the swelling and help shape it so that it could be placed into the socket of an above-knee prosthesis.

Patients who have an amputation done below the knee can learn to walk without a noticeable limp, but patients with above-knee prostheses have a noticeable gait. The artificial knee mechanism used in the prosthesis gives the gait a more mechanical cadence compared to a normal knee. I had her fitted with a prosthesis after everything had healed and was painless. I had her followed by a specialist in physical medicine and rehabilitation at Madison General Hospital because of his expertise with pediatric amputees. I never saw her after that first year, and as she outgrew each of her prostheses, the physiatrist had her fitted with a new one.

Six or seven years later, while I was at the Dean Clinic, she saw Dr. Walter Baranowski, who had replaced me at the East Madison Clinic, for an orthopedic problem unrelated to her amputation. He asked her why she had decided to see him rather than me since I had saved her life. She told him she would never see me again because I had taken off her leg. You can imagine how disappointed I felt to hear that from him, but I believe I can understand how sometimes it is important to find someone you can blame for a disability that has caused you considerable anguish. We see this often when women sue their obstetricians after they have delivered an imperfect child through no fault of their doctor's.

My interest in the surgical management of severely disabled patients with rheumatoid arthritis and especially their hand problems dates back to my residency, where I was given the responsibility as chief resident to oversee the weekly hand conferences. Since there is an overlap in orthopedic hand surgery and plastic surgery, I was able to persuade the plastic surgery residents to participate in our conference to make it more useful for both disciplines. I carried this with me while at Sheppard Air Force Hospital, because none of the other surgeons had much interest in hand cases. A significant percentage of the patients we treated were retirees, and a number had advanced rheumatoid arthritis so that it was possible to help them using the various corrective procedures I had been trained to perform. Drs. Sundstrom, Harrington, and Hirsch were pleased that I had this interest. There were not many orthopedic surgeons in Madison who had much interest or experience in the use of artificial joints made of a rubbery plastic known as Silastic. These small implants were designed for use in the hand, particularly the knuckles, known as MCP joints.

Over time, rheumatoid arthritis can ravage the joints of the hands, and while I reconstructed the hands of a great number of rheumatoid arthritics during my career, one patient stands out. She had been under the care of a rural family doctor who had been a fatalist as far as surgical benefits were concerned for this condition. This attitude resulted in both of her hands and wrists deteriorating until they became almost useless stumps. When Dr. Sundstrom first saw her, he thought I could probably help her but was not certain how, given her degree of disability. Both of her wrists had been so destroyed by the arthritis that her hands had fallen off at a forty-five degree angle to the sides of the wrists, giving rise to the designation of an opera-glass hand. The configuration of the hands themselves took on the appearance of mittens with undersized thumbs that were almost plastered to her palms.

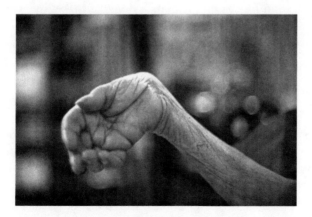

Figure 11 Opera-glass hand from rheumatoid arthritis

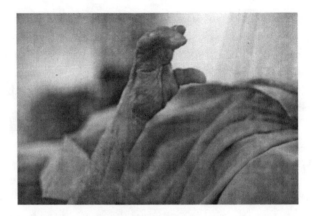

Figure 12 Opera-glass hand post-op wrist and knuckle surgery

She could not hold anything in either hand and would pick up objects using both of her wrists. She could hardly dress herself, and her footwear consisted of slippers. I did not know it at the time, but her husband, who had a drinking problem, was often abusive to her. My goal was to stabilize her wrists by fusing the remaining bones of her wrist and placing her hands in a centralized position. I did this by taking bone graft from her pelvis and placing it in a trough I made in the bones that made up her wrist. In addition, I placed a large pin through her third metacarpal bone (long bone located in the palm) and into the main wrist bone, known as the radius. It took a couple of months to heal, and then I put in Silastic joints in the knuckles and fused the finger joints in a functional position. A functional position for the finger joints is one that makes the hand look like it is about to catch a ball. With the thumb now out and her palm and the fingers basically motored by the knuckle joints, she could now oppose her thumb and index finger and get her hand around a glass, which allowed her to drink and eat more normally.

While this whole undertaking took four sessions in the operating room, she was dramatically transformed both physically and psychologically. She changed from a depressed woman who tried to hide her hands to someone who smiled and had regained some pride. Over the years, she allowed me to replace her knees and hips, and I am certain that if anyone said prayers on my behalf she was one of them. Actually, I feel blessed to have been given the opportunity to make a big difference in her life. I would not have had the technology available to make this happen if I had been in practice thirty or forty years earlier.

Another of the challenging cases illustrated in figures 13, 14, 15, and 16 was a woman whose knuckle joints, known as the metacarpophalangeal joints, were so damaged that the fingers deviated at a forty-five degree angle along with a thumb that took on the appearance of a duckbill. By replacing these joints with prostheses and balancing the muscles and tendons that control the joints, along with thumb reconstruction, it was possible to create a very functional and cosmetically improved hand. The same is seen in the patient whose picture shows a pre-op and post-op reconstruction that allowed her to hold a glass of water, a task she previously could not do with one hand.

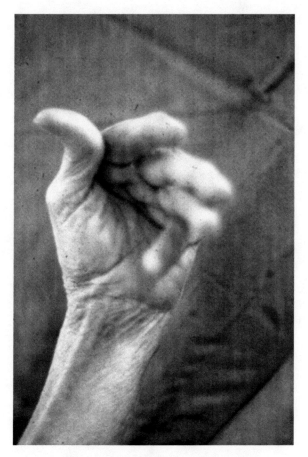

Figure 13 Palm view of severe rheumatoid hand

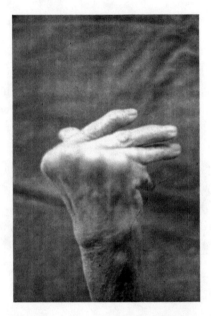

Figure 14 Back view of severe rheumatoid hand

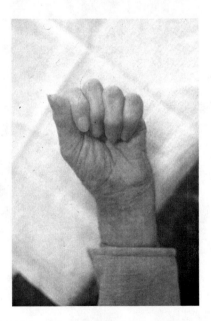

Figure 15 Palm view post-op knuckle joint replacements and tendon realignments

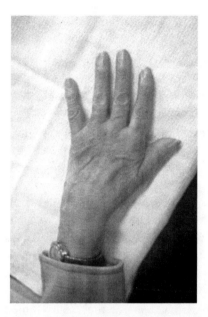

Figure 16 Back view of reconstructed rheumatoid hand

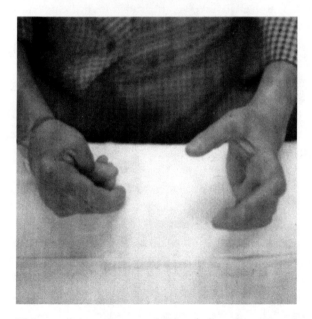

Figure 17 Pre-op right and post-op left hand of another severe rheuma-toid hand

One of the best things that happened to me in my first several years of practice was to have been in a clinic (EMC) that had an outstanding rheumatologist. He was just as outstanding as a human being. Dr. Walter Sundstrom had no peers outside of the university in private practice in Madison, which at that time had three major multispecialty clinics, as well as a great number of single specialty groups, family practice groups, and solo practitioners. Because I was the primary orthopedic surgeon for the EMC, I developed a large population of arthritis patients who needed reconstructive surgery varying from joint replacements, joint fusions, and tendon transfers. I took as many courses as possible in reconstructive procedures at various centers located in Boston, New York, Atlanta, Los Angeles, San Francisco, Chicago, and Salt Lake City to name a few. At about the same time, I left the EMC and joined the Dean Clinic, Dr. Sundstrom joined the internal medicine department at University Hospital, where he eventually became a full professor and chair of the rheumatology section. During the first several years of his tenure there, Dr. Sundstrom continued to send me surgical cases.

Shortly after I started practicing at the Dean Clinic, the internal medicine department there hired their own rheumatologist, Dr. Tim Harrington, who had came from a Texas university involved in academic medicine and was now going into private practice with a multispecialty group. Like Dr. Sundstrom, Dr. Harrington was an excellent clinician. He was drawn back to Madison where he had grown up and where his father still lived. We got along very well professionally and personally and went on fishing trips along with several others from the clinic to a beautiful chain of lakes in northern Wisconsin.

While Dr. Harrington tried to distribute his referrals fairly among the members of the Dean Clinic orthopedic department, he tended to refer me some of the more complex cases, in part because he knew I enjoyed the challenge. There were a number of patients with such severe rheumatoid arthritis that they had been confined to wheelchairs for several years before seeing Dr. Harrington. This often happened when their family doctor had told them there was not much more that could be done for them. One such patient was Sophie Moen, who actually came to me from Dr. Tom Hirsch, also an excellent clinician and very compassionate specialist. He was the second rheumatologist hired by the Dean Clinic after Dr. Harrington's arrival. The patient, who was referred to Dr. Hirsch from a rural community, had been in a wheelchair for over five years and her body configuration had taken on the appearance of the wheelchair. She had developed joint contractures in her hips and knees that prevented her limbs from straightening out.

Her husband, who was her caretaker, had to lift her from her bed into the wheelchair in the morning, on to the toilet when necessary, and back into bed at night. When he began to have back problems because of all the lifting, they were referred to Dr. Hirsch for advice on what more could be done for her. He told them that unless she could learn to walk and become more independent that she would likely have to go to a nursing home, which did not sit well with either of them. When he told her he thought I might be able to replace her severely damaged hips and knees and release her contractures, they both opted to see me about that possibility.

When I first saw Mrs. Sophie Moen, she could not have weighed more that 120 pounds, which in retrospect was good because it would result in less stress on any artificial joint replacements that involved weight-bearing joints. Her X-rays showed typical changes of advanced rheumatoid arthritis with complete loss of joint space, indicating the cartilage was gone. The X-rays also showed advanced osteoporosis in her bones from a combination of lack of weight-bearing stress and the cortisone drugs she had previously taken.

I spent a considerable amount of time not only explaining the nature of the artificial joints, made at that time from a combination of metal and plastic materials, but also emphasized the arduous rehabilitation she would have to endure, particularly since she had been wheelchair bound for so long. One thing that was in her favor was that because patients with rheumatoid arthritis suffer with so much pain for so long they develop a pain tolerance that is significantly higher compared to someone with osteoarthritis and single joint involvement.

One postoperative complication that is unique with patients like Sophie Moen is that they frequently get stress fractures in their osteoporotic bones once they start to become ambulatory, so it is necessary to go very slowly when it comes time to get them into a standing position much less even walking. In her case I used a tilt table that allowed her to be supine initially, and then I would tilt the table to various degrees, which elevated the head of the table until the patient eventually tolerated the standing position. We started at about forty-five degrees of elevation for fifteen minutes at a time and increased the time and degrees until she could tolerate the fully upright position without bone pain in her thighs or legs.

We decided to do one joint at a time because I did not think she could tolerate having both knees or both hips or one knee and one hip done under the same anesthetic. We did the knees first. When she was in the hospital for her third joint, which was the left hip, and was recovering well from this surgery, her husband, who was returning home from visiting her in the hospital, had a heart attack while driving his car and died. Sophie had no choice other than to go to a nursing home when she was discharged from the hospital after about a ten-day stay.

Three months after her husband died, she was back in the hospital for her last joint replacement, which went as well as her previous three. We talked about what a blessing in disguise her decision to proceed with her surgeries had been. Had her husband died before any of her surgeries were done, it probably would have insured her lifelong confinement to a nursing home. Now she knew she was only going to be there as long as it took to learn to walk on her own.

As expected, she did develop a minor stress fracture in the tibia of her right leg, but this healed uneventfully. She left the nursing home, using a walker for assistance initially. Gradually she was able to walk with a cane and finally, just over a year from her first surgery, she was walking independently. A family member recounted how each Sunday before her surgeries her husband would roll her wheelchair down the center aisle to the pew in the front of their church in rural Wisconsin. The first time she walked down that aisle after her husband's death, all those in attendance stood up and applauded, many with tears in their eyes. It is stories like this that make the practice of medicine so fulfilling. Despite her loss, I could see the happiness and almost reverence in her face every time she came in for a follow-up visit to my office.

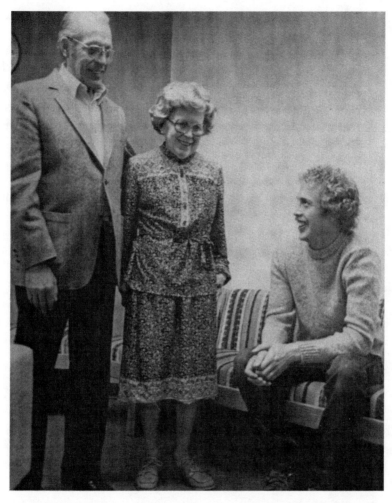

Figure 18 Sophie Moen with brother and nephew shortly after regaining
ability to walk

This next patient referred to me by Dr. Sundstrom represents an example of a positive personal relationship that doctors can develop with their patients. I think it is generally wise not to become attached emotionally, as it may interfere with your judgment. In the case of Marion Brown, it was a friendship based on an understanding of each other's personal characteristics. She was one of the most intelligent and warmhearted persons I had ever met. She was trained as a biochemist, just as her husband Wayne had been; only she apparently was a much better student.

She told me how after they had graduated from the university, gotten married, and were working, there had been an opening for a position in the Wisconsin State Laboratory of Hygiene for a head biochemist. They both applied, but Wayne got the job. She said she knew he was going to get the job. There was very little opportunity for women to get leadership roles in that field, particularly if competing against a man for the same job in state government. She never held it against Wayne but was never shy about telling people the story about it. She eventually started raising a family of wonderful children who I came to know over the years.

Dr. Sundstrom introduced us when it became apparent that the arthritis in her hip had advanced to the point where she no longer wanted to live with that degree of disability. Total joint replacements had just recently become available in this country after Sir John Charnley developed some of the first in England. The technology had been developed about the time I was going into the Air Force in 1969.

When I entered practice in Madison, I had not yet done a total joint replacement but had taken courses on the technique, which was similar in many ways to replacing a femoral head or the ball side of the hip that for years we had been doing for broken hips. It was also similar to a cup arthroplasty, an operation that involves putting a stainless steel cup in the hip socket for arthritis. It was just a matter of becoming familiar with the instruments and implants (plastic sockets and a stemmed metal ball). I had the opportunity to watch my friend, Dr. Andrew McBeath, do a couple, and felt comfortable in being able to do them myself. My partner, Dr. Blair, and I would assist one another to give ourselves additional experience. Marion Brown was one of my first patients for that procedure. The operation went very well, and she was extremely happy to be free of her pain.

Marion liked to know as much about her doctors as they would allow her to know, and before long she knew the names of my wife and children. I always tried to spend a little extra time with her, even when I was running late. We would talk about everything from family to politics. I learned when making post-op rounds to see her last, especially when she came in to have her other hip done several years later. This way if I had a little extra time I would spend it with her and if I was running late I could use that as an excuse to get to the office or home to see my family. After her second surgery, when she would come in for a post-op follow-up, we would greet each other with a kiss as her husband stood by and watched. I believe he actually enjoyed it. Later Wayne became a patient of mine for his chronic back ailment, a problem that fortunately did not require surgery.

About ten years after Marion's second hip replacement, she fell asleep on a couch, got up wrong, and dislocated her second hip. This is always a shock to a patient, because the hip goes from being painless to one they have no control over and movement of any type is painful. She was taken to St. Mary's emergency room, where I met her, reviewed her X-rays, and told her I would try to put it back in place in the emergency room by giving her a muscle relaxant and pain-killer intravenously. If I could not get it back in this way, I would have to take her to the operating room to attempt another manipulation to put it back in place or with open surgery. Fortunately, I succeeded in putting it back in place in the emergency room, kept her in the hospital overnight, and sent her home with a brace to use at night and crutches to walk on for a week. As it turns out, every couple of years for the next several years the same thing would happen, and each time we succeed in getting it back in place in the emergency room.

At one point, I briefly discussed trying to do something surgical to prevent this from happening. She was approaching ninety, and we both decided it would not be a wise choice. I saw her in follow-up annually. Our families became good friends, and we had dinner with them at their retirement center and had them to our house for the same. Marion knew I liked to write opinions and was an occasional guest editorial writer in the Madison newspapers. She also knew that they would not publish me more than once a month, so when she learned I wrote many more opinions than were published she asked if I would e-mail them to her, which I did for years. Her daughter later told me she saved the ones that were published in a scrapbook.

Marion had decided at one point she would like to give money in the form of stocks to the University of Wisconsin medical school and asked me if I would give her a suggestion about how the money should be earmarked. Based on my personal needs and heritage as a medical student, I told her that I thought the idea of a scholarship given to a first-generation American in need of financial help would be my choice. She thought this was a great idea, and her funds went toward establishing that type of scholarship.

When Marion Brown and husband began to falter because of their age, they decided to enter a nursing home together in Janesville, about thirty miles south of Madison, where her daughter and son-in-law lived. By that time, I had already retired but would go down to see them about once a year. Wayne died about a year or so before Marion. He was cremated, and his ashes were saved and buried with Marion, who did not want to be cremated. I attended her funeral and burial, which I found moving, especially hearing her daughter and friends talk about my dear friend and patient. She was someone I had admired and learned to love. When she died, it was like closing a chapter of my life.

One last patient, David Slautterback, PhD, whom I would like to mention from my years of private practice, was a professor in the anatomy department at the University of Wisconsin medical school. His area of expertise was in microscopic anatomy, more specifically with the electron microscope, which allowed scientists to observe the structures inside of cells of the body invisible to the naked eye.

When I was a medical student, he was relatively new to the faculty. He had been given responsibility for the electron microscope lab. During Dr. Slautterback's career, he was responsible for the development and techniques that made the university one of the leaders in this field of research. Like Dr. Mortenson, the chairman of the department of anatomy, he was very laid-back and kind. He was not only a remarkably bright person but also very generous with his time. From when I was a first-year medical student until the next time I had any personal contact with him, almost thirty years had passed. He had not changed one iota, and I was humbled by the fact that he had come to see me about the increasing disability he was having from advanced osteoarthritis of his hips. I was not certain he remembered me, as it had been thirty years since I had him as a teacher. It is certainly difficult for me to remember specific details about the majority of the patients I have only seen in the office and not in surgery after thirty years.

I did not ask him how he came to be referred to me, as I was more interested in seeing what it was that I could do for him. As I had done for all of the patients I have seen with X-ray evidence of advanced osteoarthritis, I advised him we would not be treating his X-ray but the degree of disability the arthritis was causing him. We see some patients who have horrible-looking X-rays that produce minimal symptoms and some who have mild to moderate changes on X-ray that cause considerable pain and limited movement of the hip.

After deciding whether a patient has had a fair trial of conservative treatment, which in the case of the hip includes various anti-inflammatory medications, physical therapy, reduction of painful activities, and the use of a cane, crutches, or walker, I would discuss what surgery entails. It was not only important to tell patients what a hip replacement consisted of as far as the implants are concerned, but what the complications and risks of the procedure could be. I invariably told them whether I thought they were a candidate for the procedure. If I thought they were a good candidate, I would tell them that they would determine the timing of the procedure based on whether they no longer wanted to live with their degree of disability and pain.

Before patients would finally decide to proceed, it was important to define clearly what they should expect in terms of relief of pain and physical activities. Despite commercials on television and advertisements in newspaper and magazines or what their friends may tell them, an artificial joint still has certain inherent limitations. This is true in the newer metal on metal hips and even those using surface replacement technologies. I had the good fortune to provide Dr. Slautterback with two new hips over a period of a few years, and he was an ideal patient.

I have met many people who have left a lasting impression. One of those is a pediatrician whom I have gotten to know more personally in retirement than during my years of practice. He was actually near the end of his active career by the time I joined the Dean Clinic. He had been the first pediatrician to join the clinic and had recruited several others, including his younger brother. This team made a very strong and vibrant pediatric department. My first exposure to him was as a medical student on a pediatric rotation at St. Mary's Hospital.

The pediatric service at this hospital had a significant number of inpatients, in great part due to the busy practices of the Dean Clinic pediatricians, led by Dr. Tom Geppert. As a result, the UW medical school saw this hospital pediatric service as an important part of their mission to provide medical students with an excellent education. Dr. Geppert was a remarkable teacher with what appeared to have been a photographic memory. When we would make rounds, he would pause at each bed to point out salient physical findings and important parts of the patient's history. With each disorder, he would refer to a particular medical journal by name, date, and often page that contained useful information regarding the disorder. When a seriously ill child came in with meningitis one day, he showed us how to perform a spinal tap on a child, which he did with the dexterity of a skilled surgeon.

The Dean pediatricians took care of a large percentage of the babies and children the University of Wisconsin Hospital interns and residents had while they were still in training, including my own children. It was not until years after Tom retired that I learned that the Dean Clinic consulting accountant had called him on the carpet for all the free care he had been providing. According to Tom, the clinic accountant, Oscar Gaarder, visited him one day and told him he had cost the clinic thirty-five thousand dollars in fees and lab work with all of his "no charges" the previous year. He informed Mr. Gaarder that all his patients from Maple Bluff (high-income residential area) were able to get appointments to see him whenever they wanted. Until he received complaints that they could not, he saw no reason to change his practice of not charging poor patients or those in special groups. Actually, when I joined the clinic, it was also customary to make no office charges for seeing members of the clergy, other doctors, and their family members.

Many years later one of the mothers of Tom's patients, whose nine children Tom had treated, sent him a picture of her family after they had grown up. She mentioned that four of them had earned doctorates. Along with the picture, she indicated to Dr. Geppert that she was very aware that his one-dollar charge for each of their visits to the clinic was supposed to have been much more and that she greatly appreciated all he had done for them. While Tom has not seen patients for years, he continues to keep up with the pediatric literature. At the same time, he is making grandfather clocks, furniture, and watercolor and oil paintings, along with playing golf, as he approaches his ninetieth birthday. Whoever developed the Energizer bunny concept obviously knew Dr. Tom Geppert.

The cost of medical care, even when the charges for an office visit back in the forties were only a few dollars, could be a real hardship on people, particularly large families. The elderly were often not charged anything by a large percentage of doctors if it was obvious they could not afford the customary fees at that time. When Medicare became a reality, many physicians who had provided this free care were finally compensated.

As I understand it, the majority of doctors were first opposed to Medicare. They looked upon it as a government intrusion, but some soon learned that they were earning more because of being compensated for what had been previously charity care. As medical technology progressed to permit innumerable diagnostic tests and revolutionary procedures like organ transplants, cardiac revascularization, artificial joint replacements, and endoscopic procedures to repair hernias, ligaments, cartilage, and so forth, the cost of medical care has skyrocketed—to the point where even private insurers are now balking at paying full price. As a result, health maintenance organizations, preferred provider groups, private insurers, and others have negotiated with medical providers to pay only a percentage of customary fees. It has gotten to the point where hardly any payer now pays full price. Medicaid pays about 45 to 50 percent of usual and customary charges; Medicare pays 80 percent of the charges that existed five or more years ago; and other third party payers like HMOs pay from 75 to 80 percent of the charges.

Many large clinics have become top-heavy with administrative people. Consequently, when belt-tightening occurs because of higher costs and lower reimbursements, they are some of the first to be let go. One experience that I had with the administrative people I dealt with before retiring had to do with a limitation of charges I had put on the brother of one of my medical school classmates. This patient, who lived over two hundred miles north of Madison, never would have come to the Dean Clinic for his surgery if he had not been recommended to me by his brother. He needed a total knee replacement for severe degenerative arthritis. I knew the patient because I had a northern Wisconsin vacation home near his hometown. I had examined his knees a number of times over the years when on vacation at the request of my classmate Dr. David Pierpont.

His brother had health insurance, but it had a reputation of not paying well. So when he asked me to do his surgery I agreed to do it as an insurance-only case. This way he would not have any out-of-pocket expenses for what his insurance did not pay. His wife stayed at our home during his hospitalization.

When I discharged him from the hospital, he also stayed with us for a few days while my wife, a physical therapist, worked with him on his exercises. A few weeks later, I got a call from an administrator in the billing department. He stated I was not going to be allowed to treat the patient as insurance only because the clinic could get in trouble for doing so. Hearing this and being aware of all of the discounts that were given to various payers annoyed me. I argued with him, and he finally relented. However, he said the difference in collection of my charges as well as the anesthesiologist charges would be subtracted from my bookings for the month. I pointed out to him that there was no way this patient would have ever come to the Dean Clinic if it had not been for my friendship with his brother. Reluctantly, I agreed to accept this compromise, despite the fact that before this incident discounts went into clinic overhead costs shared by all the members of the clinic rather than just by one.

In January of 1996, two years before I retired, my reflections for that new year concerning pain and medical care were published in the St. Mary's Hospital medical staff newsletter that is sent to all staff once a month. Those thoughts were as follows:

The pain our patients experience comes in many forms:

- As the gnarled, swollen, stiff, rheumatoid hand that attempts to button a shirt;

- As the tender breast lump and its associated anxiety;

- The searing back pain from collapsing brittle vertebrae;

- Occluding coronaries forcing the core of our being to hunger for oxygen;

- The kidney stone that doubles up its victim with knifelike punishment;

- The sorrow in the eyes of the mother whose child is withering away from a relentless malignancy;

- The multiple vague pains of the woman whose husband is a philanderer;

In treating these, as well as the many other forms of pain, we have at our disposal the many advances of technology—computers, radiation, surgery, laser treatments, endoscopy, and various pharmacologic remedies. Yet, these alone are all devoid of the element of care that ultimately helps fulfill the needs of these patients. It is the genuinely expressed compassion and concern that we are able to show our patients as we hold their hands when necessary, make eye contact, allow them to cry on our shoulders, and at times even share our own tears with them.

Lesson 14 (a):
Become a Volunteer—My African Experience

When I decided to retire in January 1998, I was able to get off the night-call schedule a year before my scheduled date of retirement. Two senior orthopedic surgeons in our department asked the members of our department to get off the night call schedule. Life in medicine becomes quite a bit easier if you do not have to go to the hospital for emergencies at all hours of the day and night. Emergencies no longer interrupt your clinic schedule. Patients with scheduled appointments do not have to wait for you to get back from the hospital or for you to do an urgent procedure in the clinic, like repairing a laceration or draining an abscess of a finger or limb. Our orthopedic department agreed that after the one year of "no call", if we wanted to stay on at the clinic as nonoperating orthopedic surgeons, we would be allowed to do that. While my senior partners had decided to do exactly that for a few years, I thought I would prefer to quit private practice at or near the peak of my surgical skills to avoid the "Dr. First Syndrome."

I also wanted to do some volunteer work in the Third World at some time and thought this would be a good time to do it. Orthopedics Volunteer Overseas (OVO) was an organization that had an information booth at all of the annual Academy of Orthopedic Surgeons Society meetings that I regularly attended. I saw pictures of the kind of work they were doing with patients, but even more importantly, I could see that they spent considerable time teaching orthopedic surgery to doctors and medical assistants that allowed them to do things for their own people when the volunteers were not there. The mother organization that OVO was a part of is called Health Volunteers Overseas (HVO). This organization includes physical therapists, dentists, nurses, and medical doctors in specialties like pediatrics, internal medicine, plastic surgery, hand surgery, urology, and orthopedic surgery.

Ever since reading a biography of Dr. Albert Schweitzer when I was a premed student, I thought it would be gratifying to follow in his steps. I chose an African

117

country as the part of the world where I would go to do surgery and teach. Specifically I chose Tanzania, located on the east coast of Africa, just south of Kenya. The application process was similar to requirements made of doctors applying for hospital privileges in this country's major metropolitan areas. This includes curriculum vitae with copies of one's bachelor's degree, medical degree, internship and residency certificates, medical license, board certification, hospital privileges, malpractice experience, and at least two letters of reference from colleagues who were familiar with your practice. All of this information was done in duplicate, because it was not unheard of for everything getting lost somewhere in transit between the United States and the country you were going to do your volunteer work. Most of the sites required a month. Travel expenses, food, and housing were all paid by volunteers, so it ends up costing several thousand dollars for one person and more, of course, if you take your spouse.

Fortunately, Barb felt the same way I did about sharing our knowledge and skills with people who desperately needed it. While she had retired almost two years before I had, she kept her license current, accompanied me, and worked at the same hospital. Her area of special interest is physical therapy for children with physical and developmental disabilities. Over the years, she had taken continuing education classes that allowed her to acquire knowledge and skills necessary to help pediatric patients in this particular problem area. She had been employed for about fifteen years at the Central Wisconsin Center for the Developmentally Disabled. As one might expect, there was a great need for her at the hospital, since neither of the two physical therapists there had any special training in this area.

The Bugando Hospital in Mwanza, Tanzania, located at the southern shore of Lake Victoria, was built in the 1970s and was the site of my assignment. An eight-hundred-bed hospital was built with money raised by the Roman Catholic bishops of Germany. This same group hired European doctors in most specialties to staff the hospital and was responsible for their salaries as well as providing homes for them. After about ten years, the German Catholic bishops turned the responsibility of the hospital to the Tanzanian government and the bishop of Tanzania. As one could imagine, neither had adequate funds to cover the costs, and it was not long before the hospital lost its European specialists and began to deteriorate physically. In some of the specialty areas, a few African doctors had joined the hospital staff and had remained after the Europeans left. They included two general surgeons, a couple of pediatricians, internists, and an anesthesiologist.

Even now, there are only ten fully trained doctors to serve the needs of eight million people. The Bugando Hospital (Bugando) was the only resource they had for Western medicine. At the time of our assignment in 1998, there was only one medical school in all of Tanzania, with its population of about twenty-nine million, and it was located in Dar es Salaam. In America, there is one doctor for every four hundred patients; whereas in Tanzania there is one for every twenty-five thousand. Quite a few of the Tanzanian doctors were trained in Russia, which had been trying to gain influence in this part of the world. In fact, the doctor I was training in orthopedic surgery had gone to medical school in Russia.

Bugando had no way of meeting the medical needs of the people it served, and thus was a treasure trove of pathologic conditions and needy people who volunteer and missionary organizations could help and learn from. One such organization, the Maryknoll missionaries, had sent a doctor who was also a priest, Peter Le Jacq, there in the 1980s. When he arrived, there was no running water, irregular electricity, and essentially no bedding. According to people we met who knew him well, Dr. Le Jacq found he was gagging from the odor that permeated the hospital. The odor was created by the lack of functioning toilets and insufficient electricity to keep bodies frozen in the hospital morgue. He was reportedly the son of a wealthy New York financier, so he called home to talk to his father about sending him money to make the changes needed to make it tolerable for people to work there. Because of his and others' efforts, enough money was raised to construct a small hydroelectric power plant, a rudimentary plumbing system complete with water pumps, and a pipeline directly from Lake Victoria.

Le Jacq, who obtained his medical education at Cornell before becoming a priest, epitomizes the American volunteer or missionary who goes to a Third World country to give. He is often quoted as saying that if there is a heaven, he did not need to live comfortably in this world. He apparently figured he would have all eternity to be comfortable if he did what Jesus said for him to do, which was to sell what he had and give it to the poor. He apparently felt that part of what he had to give away was his Cornell education. He certainly represents a modern-day Albert Schweitzer in my mind. From what I have learned from a physician who actually knew Dr. Schweitzer, Le Jacq had a much softer veneer. Perhaps having French as opposed to a German ancestry may have played a role.

Our trip to Tanzania took twenty-six hours with a plane change in Amsterdam plus an overnight stay in Dar es Salaam, Tanzania. The flight from Dar es Salaam took only a few hours, and, upon our arrival at the Mwanza airport, we were picked up by a Tanzanian driver who was employed by the Maryknoll mission where we were going to stay during our time in Mwanza. The road from the airport to the city had once been blacktop but was now a potholed, dusty, gravel road. There were certainly not as many vehicles as one would expect in an area with a population of several million people. Most of the buildings in the city were no more than three stories high, with the exception of a couple of hotels. Most of the men we saw on our way to the hospital wore ordinary Western shirts and pants. Many of the women wore colorful wraparounds that allowed them to carry their children.

The house owned by the Maryknolls was one of several that had been built for the construction workers who had come to Africa to build the hospital in the 1970s. It was a concrete block construction with three bedrooms, two showers, a dining area, and a library with a computer in it. The computer was a godsend, as it allowed us to communicate with family and friends back in the United States. We had no television and only a short-range portable radio. We were not able to get much current news or information without going to the main hotel where there was a television or by using the computer. Unfortunately, there was a fair amount of demand for computer time, and we were encouraged to limit our use of it to not more than an hour or so because of costs per week for the Maryknolls.

There were two others sharing the house with us, and both were anesthesiologists. The senior of the two was Ray O'Brian from Ireland, who belonged to an organization that was the equivalent of our Peace Corps. He had had a few other previous assignments in Africa, in which he had functioned both as a family doctor and as an anesthesiologist before coming here. He had been at Bugando for about five years and was a great resource of information. The other anesthesiologist, Dr. Tom Fell, was in private practice with a large single specialty group in Olympia, Washington; they allowed him to take time off to do volunteer work. His father had also been a doctor who had done volunteer work in Madagascar, an island off the southeastern coast of Africa. When he was a boy, Tom had accompanied him a number of times.

The Bugando Hospital had a program for teaching nurse anesthetists. Ray had taken the primary responsibility for the program, but Dr. Tom Fell was also a very able teacher. Tom brought with him anesthesia equipment that he donated to the hospital. A vast majority of the equipment at the hospital and in particular on the orthopedic service had been donated from outside of Africa. Virtually all of the orthopedic instruments, implants like rods, screws, plates, intramedullary nails, and metallic prostheses had come from the United States, from volunteers like me. This also included surgical patient drapes, an air-powered drill, and a portable X-ray machine, the last two of which were inoperable during my assignment period. There was no one there with technical knowledge who could repair them, much less have the available parts necessary to replace if needed.

In America, many of the things we use in orthopedics are disposable items like plates, screws, and other hardware. In Africa, if any such implant is removed, it is cleaned and then put back on the shelf to be used again in another patient. Some of the implants, like rods, for example, have the length and diameter etched at one end of each rod, but in many instances they had been used so many times, one could no longer read the size of the rod. Drill points were similarly reused, and almost all of them were dull, resulting in the surgeon being virtually drenched with perspiration by the end of each operation from laboring with these manual tools. Sterile paper drapes were used for most cases that involved significant bleeding, but they were in low supply most of the time. Most of the sterile linen drapes used in surgery were about a third of the size used in America, so that often two or more had to be used to cover the patient adequately. Most of the linen drapes had two or more patches on them with an occasional hole still not patched.

The operating room dedicated to orthopedic surgery was as large as most operating rooms in the States; however, the overhead lighting left a lot to be desired. The hospital was not air-conditioned, but the orthopedic room had a small window air conditioner that provided some relief when the outside temperature was in the nineties. Fortunately, all the rooms were supported by an auxiliary generator should the hospital lose its electricity; that happened a number of times during my time there. In fact, at least once a week we would be without electricity for several hours in the house we lived in, and if it happened after sundown we went to bed early and used flashlights to read or to find the bathroom.

When I came to Bugando in 1998, I was one of nine orthopedic surgeons who were assigned a month each to the hospital to teach Dr. Dass, a first-generation African, by doing surgery, holding outpatient clinics, and giving lectures. The beauty of having nine qualified people follow one another was that complex orthopedic problems could be properly managed. Knowing there would soon be someone fully trained to see the patient in follow-up after each assignment was completed made managing complex cases more comfortable. The other important aspect of having expert surgeons follow one another was that there would be a qualified person there to manage problems, particularly if a complication should occur. In addition to Dr. Dass, we were responsible for an X-ray teaching conference for the physician assistants. Upon completion of their training, most of these people were sent out into the rural areas. They were the sole source of medical attention for some of the small towns or villages. Frequently they had to compete with the tribal witch doctors for the patients' care.

After WWI, Tanzania, known as German East Africa, became a British Mandate and was renamed Tanganyika. It was during that time that Dr. Dass's father, who was a physician in India employed by the British government, came to Africa. He settled in the town of Mwanza where he brought his wife and raised his family. Dr. Dass did his undergraduate work at a university in Dar es Salaam, now the nation's capital. Because of a lack of political influence, he did not get into the medical school there and instead went to medical school in Russia. Dass pointed out that wealthier students with poorer grades were more apt to get into medical school because of bribes paid to key people with influence in the medical school.

Dass indicated that he went to Russia with a number of Tanzanian students. There they were each assigned to a Russian student who lived with them and was responsible for overseeing their activities. He indicated whenever they watched television news about America they only saw union strikes and political rallies against the U.S. government. In addition, most of what he saw about Africa depicted half-naked savages killing innocent people. He judged from seeing the African news in Russia that the American news was also a complete distortion of reality. He indicated that one of his fellow students struck up a relationship with a department store clerk. After he started dating her, the KGB visited him and told him that he should avoid seeing her again because she was a prostitute. The student did not believe them and continued seeing her, only to be taken to a mental hospital where he was drugged to the point of becoming an incoherent zombie. After a few weeks of this, Dr. Dass and his classmates contacted their embassy about the situation. Fortunately, the student was rescued and sent back to Tanzania.

In general, Tanzania was a safe country for Americans to do volunteer work. It had gained its independence from Britain in 1961 and became a socialist country with relatively peaceful people. Their only major conflict occurred in the 1970s when Idi Amin attempted to annex a northern province; this led Tanzania to go to war with Uganda until the Tanzanian army, with the help of Ugandan and Rwandan guerrillas, forced Amin to leave. About one third of the population is Christian, one third Muslim, and the remainder of various tribal or traditional beliefs. In Mwanza, the most prominent building was the hospital, which was built on the top of an elevation overlooking the poorest section of the city. The next most prominent building was the mosque, located in the downtown or business district; it had a large white dome that could be seen from afar. We often walked past it on our way into town, which was about a mile or so from our house. The call to prayer for the Muslims became a familiar sound for us and echoed throughout the surrounding area. It reminded me of my youth when I would hear the church bells ring before mass at our neighborhood church.

The hospital routine consisted of walking about three blocks to the hospital with Barb on most days. We had two clinic days and three operating days. The clinics consisted of a clubfoot clinic where mothers brought in their infants and children to be evaluated and treated for this congenital abnormality. This condition made the foot curl into a position in which the end and middle of the foot turned inward; the back of the foot turned under towards the opposite foot and the entire foot turned downward because of a shortened heel cord. Most of the children seen before six months of age could be treated with a corrective cast reapplied weekly, and a number would only need this form of treatment if the deformity was not severe. Children coming in over six months of age usually had casts applied to help reduce the deformity as much as possible but almost always required corrective surgery. Almost every week we had at least a couple of children on our surgery schedule with one or two clubfeet. This was one of the surgical procedures I thought we had gotten Dr. Dass to become quite proficient at doing. I particularly noticed this when I returned to Bugando in July of 2000 and saw that he made almost no mistakes and needed very little direction during this type of procedure.

The other clinic was an adult and adolescent clinic where we saw patients who frequently had spent a day or more getting to the clinic from a distant town. Unlike most clinics in America, the patients were not given appointments; all came in before the clinic opened and signed their names on a list. Dr. Dass, two physician assistants, and I saw the patients, and, if the patients didn't speak Swahili, there was usually someone there who could understand the various tribal languages.

There was an incredible number of abnormalities that I treated there seldom seen in America, but one young boy stands out above the rest because of what we were able to accomplish for him. He was thirteen years old and came to the clinic with his father. A couple of years earlier, he had gotten a serious bacterial infection in his left knee. The position of comfort for an infected knee is with the knee bent between thirty to forty degrees because of the swelling. His infection destroyed all the cartilage in his knee before it had been cured. The result was the femoral, tibial, and patellar components of his knee spontaneously fused together at about eighty degrees of bend. He apparently wasn't given crutches to walk on before it fused, and as a result he got around by duck waddling, which is to say he walked in a squatting posture that matched the degree of his knee bend. This situation kept getting worse until the left knee finally fused. The father wanted his son to be able to walk without crutches because other boys would knock him down and steal his crutches. In general, a joint that has become fused is painless, as was his knee. Over time the normal knee will deteriorate because it is being forced to bear weight in an abnormal position, and eventually this would become so painful and disabling that he would no longer be able to walk. Life in a wheelchair is an especially difficult existence in many parts of Africa due to the lack of sidewalks, ramps, and so on.

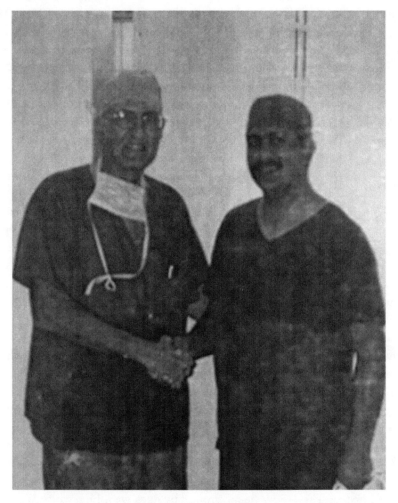

Figure 19 Dr. Dass and Dr. Pellegrino following surgery at Bugando Hospital

One of the objectives of an orthopedic training program is to teach the general principles of correcting bone and joint deformities. While I had never treated a patient in residency or in private practice with the kind of a knee problem handicapping this boy, I had treated enough deformities resulting from fractures and other congenital conditions so I knew exactly what should be done. I explained to the father and the boy that it was no longer possible to restore motion to his fused knee.

Even if total joint replacements were available in that country, he would not have been a candidate because of his age. I determined the most I could do to straighten the leg out was to remove a sizable wedge of bone from the front of the knee with the base located at the front and the apex at the back of the joint. By removing this wedge I could then close the gap, which would straighten out the leg. I realized there would be significant risk to the arteries and nerves in the back of the knee as the knee was straightened out. This was because of how much they and the other soft tissues around them had become contracted by the bent position of the knee over such a long period of time. As the knee is extended, the contracted vessels, nerves, and soft tissues are exposed to increasing tension, which can result in tearing. I informed the father and son that there was the possibility of his losing his leg if straightening the knee ended up damaging the circulation and caused gangrene. They were willing to accept this risk, so we went ahead and scheduled his surgery.

Most of the operative procedures that were done below the hip were performed under spinal anesthesia. The anesthetist inserts the needle into the space around the nerves in the spinal canal and injects an anesthetic solution to eliminate pain and the ability to move the leg for several hours if necessary. A great number of these procedures were done by the nurse anesthetists, who had become very good at performing them.

After taking photographs of his leg, a blood-pressure type of tourniquet was applied to his upper left thigh. The spinal was inserted and the leg washed with an alcohol solution followed by an antiseptic solution called provodine iodine. Sterile drapes were applied, and the leg was wrapped tightly with an elastic bandage from his toes to the tourniquet. This process removes most of the blood from the soft tissues and muscles so that once the tourniquet is elevated we can operate in a dry surgical field. This allows the surgeon to see structures much better and operate more safely. Once we elevated the tourniquet, I made a transverse incision over the front of the knee. This approach allowed me to excise the extra skin in the front of the knee that results from removing the bone wedge.

After I carefully dissected out the entire front of the knee exposing the patella, femur, and tibia, I placed an instrument, shaped a little like a pediatrician's tongue blade, which is used to examine a child's throat, immediately behind these bones. This protected the major nerves and blood vessels from being damaged by the bone-cutting instruments. Unfortunately, we did not have a power oscillating saw. Because this tool is much easier to control, I would have preferred it. Before I made the first cut I removed the patella with an instrument that is similar to a carpenter's chisel. I then carefully drilled a hole from front to back of the fused knee to determine the depth by placing an instrument called a depth gauge in the drill hole. This allowed me to determine how deep my bone cuts needed to be and gave me a fairly accurate measurement of how far I was going to advance the drill into the femur and tibia, minimizing the risk of damaging important structures. After the bone cuts were completed, I removed the wedge and slowly closed the gap until the leg was straight. I could tell that the structures in the back of the knee were getting tight as the gap was closing, so I had the anesthetist release the tourniquet to see if we could still feel a pulse in the foot. Fortunately, the pulse remained palpable, and his big toe blanched and became pink after I squeezed the end of it.

Rather than use a plate and screws to stabilize the bone cuts I had made, I decided not to use any metallic hardware in an area that had been previously infected. Instead I elected to use what is called an external fixator. This involves using two one-eighth-inch–diameter pins placed horizontally through the femur parallel to one another about six and eight inches above the osteotomy with two similar pins four and six inches below the osteotomy in the tibia. These four pins are then connected to two half-inch rods on each side of the leg with special clamps.

After we had closed the wound and put a sterile dressing on the leg, the anesthetist took the drapes down so the patient could see his leg. He said to the anesthetist in Swahili he could not believe how straight his leg looked.

The anesthetist then asked him, "Well, what do you say to your doctor?"

He looked at me and said, "*Assante sana, Doctore!*" which means, "Thank you very much, Doctor."

I could feel tears starting to well up and I replied, "*Karibu!*" which means, "You're welcome." I felt I had been amply rewarded by those simple words. The patient had to have the pins left in for eight weeks, and they were successfully removed after I had returned to the Wisconsin. Dr. Dass informed me by e-mail that he had done very well, was walking erect, and was very happy with the result of the surgery. We attempted to have him come back to the clinic when I returned for another month of teaching and surgery in July 2000, but it never worked out so that I could see him.

During my first experience at Bugando, I had dinner one evening with a Dutch surgeon who was based in Nairobi, Kenya, but traveled with the Flying Doctors organization to perform complex surgeries. These hospitals did not have doctors with the kind of training needed to perform the surgery. One such procedure involved the repair of what is called an obstetric fistula (abnormal passage) that develops when blood supply to the tissues of the vagina and the bladder (and/or rectum) is cut off during prolonged obstructed labor. This occurs when a young and small woman has a baby that is too large for the birth canal. The pressure created by the fetus pressing on the tissues causes the tissue to die, which creates a hole through which urine and/or feces pass uncontrollably.

Women who develop obstetric fistulas are often abandoned by their husbands, rejected by their communities, and forced to live an isolated existence because of the odors that accompany such a condition. This condition has disappeared for the most part in countries with a high standard of living and modern medical practices; caesarean deliveries are done for most women with cephalopelvic (baby's head and birth canal) disparity.

The Bugando Hospital did not have anyone trained in some of these very complex repairs, and the Dutch surgeon had this expertise. The hospital would line up a dozen or more cases. From seven in the morning until seven at night, he would operate for as many days as it took to finish. In our conversation over dinner, he talked about the history of this condition. One of the pioneers in developing the technique for this repair was an Australian obstetrician-gynecologist, Dr. Catherine Hamlin, and her New Zealand–born ob-gyn husband, Reginald. They had come to Ethiopia, where this condition was very common, and developed the technique that proved to be very successful. In 1974, they founded the Addis Ababa Fistula Hospital where they taught doctors from all over the world how to perform this kind of surgery. Our Dutch surgeon had gone there to learn their technique. Since its existence, the hospital has restored the lives of more than twenty-eight thousand women who would have otherwise perished or suffered lifelong complications brought on by childbirth injuries, specifically obstetric fistula.

A fascinating sidelight to this history of the doctors in Ethiopia's fistula hospital was the true story of one of the patients. She had no more than a grade school education and had gone to the hospital to have her vesico-vaginal fistula (bladder to vagina) repaired. She was so grateful for what they had done for her that she begged them to allow her to help them at the hospital. At first, she was given housekeeping duties. One day one of the partners could not assist, so she was asked to hold retractors and cut sutures. She demonstrated an aptitude for this kind of work and was eventually asked to assist in most of their procedures. After a year or so, Dr. Hamlin realized that it would be possible to teach her to perform some of the simpler procedures. Again, she showed remarkable skill, and it was not long before she was also taught how to perform complex repairs. It became evident she was performing them as well as they were able to do. She eventually became one of their best instructors, teaching others how to do what she had learned. In 1989, the Hamlins were notified that they were going to be the recipients of the Royal College of Surgeons' Honorary Gold Medal. They notified the Royal College that they would only come to receive this award if their remarkable instructor could receive one as well, and the Royal College agreed. Like the Hamlins, this Ethiopian woman has dedicated her life to helping women disabled by this terrible obstetrical complication. She appeared on the *Oprah Winfrey Show* a couple of years ago, where she received a hero's welcome.

Most of the spare time Barb and I had was spent in conversations with fellow volunteers and reading books that we had brought along as well as those in the library, where many had been donated by previous volunteers over the years. We would walk a couple of miles a day during the week. On weekends, we would walk even farther into town. We occasionally took a shortcut through the tin roof shanties where the majority of the poor people lived. The walls were made of a claylike mud that had been dried into blocks used to form the walls. Most of them had curtains rather than doors, and chickens, goats, and other small animals frequently ran in and out of some of these dwellings. Some of the homes were used to sell baked goods or trinkets to passersby. There were some open fields close to the hospital and near our residence on which children played soccer. The younger children did not use a regular soccer ball. Instead, they used a ball made from rags that had been tied together, and rolled up into a ball. In place of goalposts, they used tree branches stuck in the ground. It was fun to watch how competitive they were and how much they enjoyed what they were doing. The older boys played on a larger field with real goalposts. On Sundays, the older boys played games in uniform and with referees.

One Saturday I decided to break out a kite I brought from America. Most of the time it was not that windy, and I had to run a half block or so to get my kite up in the air. This attracted a large number of young children who seemed to enjoy seeing me fly the brightly colored kite. They may have been even more amused by seeing this six-foot-two gray-haired American running like a fool. The next day several boys were out in the same area, flying homemade kites made from newspaper, which was something I had never seen before. I was fascinated to see how well they worked.

Before we had completed our month, Barb had become personally interested in a single mother of one of her patients, a two-year-old with a progressive neurological disorder. Barb had been seeing the child a couple of times a week and was teaching the mother how to assist the child's development. The mother's name was Jacqueline. Barb had become quite fond of her two other children. The mother had completed high school and was hopeful of getting some training in hotel management from a local vocational school. Even though sending her children to school was quite inexpensive, she could hardly afford it. Barb agreed to donate approximately two hundred dollars a quarter for her children's school and for her vocational training. Rather than give the money directly to Jacqueline, Barb decided that she would ask Liz Mach, an RN and lay Maryknoll missionary, to help manage the distribution of the money. Liz worked at the hospital as the social services director, and she agreed to give Jacqueline so much a week as Jacqueline could justify the need. This worked out just fine until just before we came back for our second volunteer trip in 2000.

Jacqueline apparently started to get paranoid about Liz Mach possibly holding back money that she thought belonged to her. She became verbally abusive with people that worked with Liz, which disturbed Liz enough to decide not to act as our go-between. Because of this change, we decided our financial support should end. Jacqueline eventually got a job as a desk clerk in a hotel downtown, and her severely handicapped child succumbed to pneumonia brought on by respiratory difficulties associated with its neurological disorder. We took Jacqueline and her remaining two children out for lunch at a small outdoor pizza place. The children were dressed in their Sunday best. Jacqueline appeared to be quite appreciative of our friendship and help. We decided not to bring up the problems with treatment of Liz Mach's subordinates, and that was the last time we saw her during the remainder of our second stay.

During our second period of volunteering at Bugando, Dr. Dass had to accompany his wife to England to see a specialist about an infertility problem they were having. That was a very hectic week, but with the help of a couple of the physician assistants who could speak English I managed to make hospital rounds, do several surgeries, hold the clinics, and give the lectures and X-ray conferences without incident.

The one case that stood out among the rest that year was a life-and-death situation that rarely comes into play in orthopedics, except in major trauma cases. I saw a four-year-old boy with a high fever in addition to a swollen right knee and leg. He also had a swollen right shoulder. Blood cultures showed that he had Staph septicemia (infection in the blood). With this condition the organisms can be deposited anywhere the blood goes, including the brain and heart. He had been having leg and knee pain for a week before coming into the hospital, so it was likely they were the source of the blood infection.

I felt it was imperative to drain the sites of his infection and to start him on intravenous antibiotics before he died. He was dehydrated and looked very toxic. We started him on intravenous fluids and antibiotics as soon as we could and took him to the operating room, where I must have removed at least a quart of pus from his right leg and knee. The tibia and joint itself were involved, and the muscles overlying the tibia looked partially dead. I also incised and drained his left humerus and shoulder, and, as I was putting on the dressings, the anesthesiologist asked me to look at a soft spot on his head, which turned out to be a scalp abscess that I also drained.

Under ordinary circumstances, such a patient would go to an intensive care unit where nurse specialists would monitor him, but there was no such facility at Bugando. The best place for this kind of available supervision was actually in the recovery room. Therefore, we had him stay in recovery until it was ready to close down at the end of the afternoon. Ray, who had given the anesthesia, came back to the hospital in the middle of the night to check on him.

The next morning as I was leaving for the hospital to check in on the patient again, Ray stopped me before leaving and gave me a pint of milk to give to the boy's mother to feed her child. I knew the food rations at the hospital often were scarce so that families frequently brought food in for the patients to eat and drink. I was really moved by Ray's compassion for those he saw suffering. Sometimes the only thing provided by the hospital was tea and bananas. I was encouraged to see the boy looking better the next day, and he showed steady improvement each day thereafter.

When I returned to the States after my first trip, I prepared a talk to give to the Madison Orthopedic Society. I wanted to get others interested in going to Africa to volunteer their skills and knowledge. I also made the same presentation to both the St. Mary's Hospital and Meriter Hospital honorary staff members and to one of the local Optimist Clubs. Since my last trip two of Madison's orthopedic surgeons, Dr. Allen Breed and Dr. David Solfelt, have gone to Kenya and Uganda respectively. Both indicated they were rewarded with experiences similar to mine. After our second trip, Barb indicated to me that she did not think she could go back to Africa as a physical therapist. The work had been physically taxing on her. In addition, I think she really missed our children, who were just starting to have families of their own. I was not ready to call it quits as a volunteer orthopedic surgeon, but I decided to take it in another direction, which will be the final subject of this journey along a doctor's path.

Lesson 14 (b):
Become a Volunteer—My
American Experience

After we returned home from Tanzania in August of 2000, I took a few months off. I continued to attend and participate in the weekly orthopedic grand rounds and trauma conference at the University of Wisconsin Medical Center. Grand rounds at the UW Medical Center consist of having a faculty, fellow, or resident give a PowerPoint presentation on subjects of interest to orthopedic surgeons. They are done to update as well as expand knowledge in a specific area of orthopedics. What follows are a few presentation subjects: lower extremity deformities in children, arthroscopy of the hip, limb salvage procedures, surface replacement total hip arthroplasty, and so on. Occasionally a radiologist would be asked to present an orthopedic-related subject like three-dimensional CT scans. An ethicist might be asked to speak on child abuse as it relates to orthopedic trauma. Continuing to have contact with the residency program has always been a time of pure enjoyment for me; it also offered me an opportunity to give them an occasional historical perspective on various orthopedic subjects that some of the younger faculty members lack.

In November of 2000, I finally decided that I would like to see patients who had no insurance. This was something I had volunteered to do at the Dean Clinic. The clinic at that time provided free consultations for patients referred to us from the South Madison Community Health Clinic. This clinic saw primarily uninsured and entitlement patients who were on programs like Medicaid and BadgerCare, a state program for children. Many health-care providers and dentists in Wisconsin and throughout the country either limit or refuse to see Medicaid patients because of the low level of reimbursement.

The Dean Clinic decided to develop a community care program that was the brainchild of Jeanan Yasiri, a former local television newscaster before being hired by the clinic. One of the reasons for hiring her was that the clinic had gotten egg on its face when a mother brought her child in to be seen by the child's pediatrician. When the mother went to the reception desk to register the child, it had been noted in the computer records that this family had not paid any of their clinic bills for the past several months. The mother was asked to go to the billing department to talk to someone about the outstanding bills before the child would be seen. Instead of doing that, the mother went directly to the Madison newspapers and spoke to a reporter who created a front-page article that did not make the clinic look very compassionate.

Of course, this was an administrative policy and not the pediatrician's policy. This was the type of problems that began to occur when the clinic became large. Jeanan sent a notice to all the departments of the clinic, looking for volunteers to do free consultations on patients referred to the new community care program. Keith Kahle, one of my orthopedic partners, and I were the two in our department who agreed at that time. The program ended up with virtually all of the departments having individual doctors willing to perform this service.

My first thought was to contact the South Madison Community Health Clinic to see if they would be interested in having retired specialists like me who had kept their licenses current see patients for them in their facility. Dr. Love, a family practitioner, had initially expressed an interest in the idea, but when I later met with him and the clinic administrator, I was informed that they did not have the space, personnel, or funds to support such a group.

I then contacted one of the Dean Clinic's medical directors, Dr. Donald Logan, in the fall of 2000 about my idea, and he put me in contact with Jeanan Yasiri. My original thoughts were to organize a group of volunteers who would be allowed to use clinic offices available on medical staff's afternoons off. This would mean that the doctors at the clinic who were doing this work for nothing could concentrate on their paying patients. At the same time, the clinics would receive recognition for what the volunteers were doing.

I met with Jeanan a couple of times over the next several weeks, trying to get my idea across, and she informed me, apparently after talking to her superiors, that my idea of using clinic space was not a viable plan. She wanted me to complete my list of volunteers and then meet with her in January 2001.

During the next several weeks, I contacted between seventy and eighty doctors, most of whom were retired, to elicit their interest in this project. I explained that I thought that medicine and our community of patients had given us a good life and that by doing volunteer work for the uninsured we would be repaying society for what we had all received. I received replies from almost all of the doctors. Many gave me names of doctors that I had not yet contacted. Most of the doctors thought the idea was a great one, and approximately thirty of them said they would be interested in participating after learning more about the particulars. Most of them were concerned about malpractice coverage, since they no longer carried insurance after they were retired. Most of those that declined the invitation to volunteer had already allowed their licenses to lapse, and many had moved away from Madison. The doctors who had expressed an interest had been from the three major health providers in the area, University Physicians, Dean Clinic, and Physicians Plus. I was eventually successful in getting thirty-three firm commitments from doctors in fifteen different specialties.

While I was waiting for replies from the doctors I had sent letters to, I contacted a classmate from medical school, Dr. Haakom Carlson. Haakom had started a family-practice free clinic after he retired from his practice in Sauk-Prairie, about twenty-five miles from Madison. His clinic was held one evening a week in a local church hall for a few years until the local St. Vincent De Paul Society built a facility that housed a food kitchen, day care center, and ample space for a free medical clinic for a couple of family doctors. Their space also included a dental suite for a volunteer dentist.

Dr. Carlson was able to get the local hospital to provide free lab and X-ray services for his patients, whose incomes were no more than 180 percent of the national poverty level. In addition, his fund-raising campaign with local merchants, banks, and churches allowed his clinic to pay for their patients' prescriptions, with the patients only having to contribute one dollar for their medication. Everyone who worked with him was a volunteer. He told me about the Wisconsin State Statute that provided liability coverage at no cost to doctors who did volunteer work in a 501(c)3 (charitable) organization. Individual applications needed to be obtained from the Wisconsin Department of Administration, and each application had to be renewed annually.

The last time I met with Jeanan Yasiri, she suggested I meet with the director of the Dean Foundation, which is a 501(c)3 organization that raises funds to do clinical research projects, primarily in mental health. She put me in touch with Dr. Leslie Taylor, the medical director of the foundation, and to my delight she thought my concept was an excellent idea. She arranged for me to give a presentation to the board of directors of the foundation to elicit their support for space and funds. As I saw it, the only salaried position I thought necessary would be for the position I would call clinic coordinator, or others might call clinic manager.

In the meantime, I personally met with the CEOs of the three hospitals in Madison to ask them if they would be willing to support us by giving our patients free lab and X-rays. None of them would commit to a specific dollar amount until they had a better idea of what our needs were going to be. They informed me that it would be necessary for me to get the radiologists from their hospitals to agree to read the X-rays at no charge. I eventually got St. Mary's and Meriter Hospital radiologists to agree to perform this service for us. The Meriter cardiology group agreed to see cardiac referrals as well, since cardiology was one area we did not have covered. After meeting with the hospital CEOs individually, I met with them as a group at their request and was informed I needed to present them with a business plan before they would make their final commitment to the clinic. By that time, I had decided to call the clinic the Benevolent Specialist Project, and it has come to be known as the BSP Free Clinic.

My presentation to the Dean Foundation went very well, and they were enthusiastic in their support of the project. They agreed to provide us with a couple of examining rooms and pay for the salary and benefits of our clinic coordinator, who would essentially be considered an employee of the Dean Foundation. The position of clinic coordinator was advertised in the local paper. Dr. Leslie Taylor and I conducted the interviews together. We selected a woman, Kathy Williams, who had impressed us the most because of her excitement about the project and the fact that she had previous experience being the coordinator for a geriatric clinic at a small hospital in Stoughton, WI.

Once this was all in place, I asked my good friend and former colleague, Dr. Walter Sundstrom, if he would agree to be the medical director of the clinic. He had been retired from University Hospital's rheumatology section for a few years but remained very active in their conferences. As I have mentioned before, he had a huge mind for seeing to the details of quality medical care, and I knew that his leadership in this area would be very difficult to duplicate. He also had a great number of contacts with people at the University of Wisconsin, which helped tremendously in our getting our business plan made. He contacted a Jerry Weygandt, who was a professor and faculty member of the UW School of Business, to see if he would be willing to assist us with this task. As it turns out, Professor Weygandt had also been on the board of directors of the Dean Foundation. He made creating our business plan a project for one of his graduate students.

Dr. Sundstrom and I met on a couple of occasions with both of them to explain the details of how we expected the BSP Free Clinic to fit into the medical community. We were planning not only to serve the needs of the uninsured in the Madison area, which is Dane County, but also to be a resource for southcentral Wisconsin, which would include Sauk, Rock, Columbia, Iowa, Green, Dodge, Richland, and Jefferson counties.

Primary-care free clinics already existed in some of these counties. We were willing not only to see their patients but also patients referred to us from private individual physicians and clinics, so long as their patients met the financial criteria of eligibility of an income no greater than 180 percent of the national poverty level and were uninsured. We hoped to raise funds from individuals and organizations to help us meet our financial needs, which initially turned out to be more of a problem than we had expected.

To meet our volunteer needs I contacted a nurse, Betsy Knight, someone I had known since the late 1960s when I was a resident moonlighting at St. Mary's emergency room where she had been the head nurse. She was now a nursing supervisor for whom I had done bilateral knee replacements before retiring. Betsy gave me hospital supplies to take to Africa in both 1998 and 2000. She had been doing volunteer work in her free time at St. Martin House, which provides a free evening meal Monday through Friday for those in need in Madison. She agreed to find nurses to work in our clinic, which she succeeded in doing wonderfully well.

Once I had gotten all the completed applications from the physician volunteers, who not only had to fill out a two-page questionnaire but had to have the application notarized, I personally carried them to the state office building. There I gave them to the person responsible for getting them into the proper administrator's hands. It still took several weeks to get all of the applicants (except one) approved. The one individual, a cardiologist, had forgotten to get his license renewed a couple of years ago and therefore was not eligible to participate until that was done. Once we had gotten approval from the state, which required us to be under the 501(c)3 charter of the Dean Foundation, Meriter and St. Mary's hospitals agreed to commit five thousand dollars each for labs and X-rays. This would be determined based on what they would be normally charging for these studies. In addition, University Hospital eventually agreed to pick up the costs of two patients' hospitalizations at their facility per year should there be a need. We started seeing patients in November 2001; it had taken nearly a year for this project to become a reality. I thought it took forever while I was working with Dr. Sundstrom and Dr. Taylor to get this off the ground, but one of the hospital administrators, Jerry Leffert, later said he found it hard to believe we had accomplished so much in the time we did.

The goal of the BSP Free Clinic was to serve an unmet need brought about by our current health-care system. The majority of employed workers have health insurance as a benefit. Those individuals without jobs, particularly single mothers, are usually eligible for entitlement programs like Medicaid that pay for their medical needs. Unfortunately, many people have low-paying jobs that do not offer health insurance benefits. Consequently, the people who fall through the cracks in our current health-care system are the people we wanted to be able to help. Once again, they must meet the financial criteria of not earning more than 180 percent of the poverty level, which gets progressively higher for a married couple with children.

We function as an outpatient clinic only because our liability coverage from the State of Wisconsin does not allow us to see emergency patients, perform surgery, or admit patients to the hospital. Because all of us have practiced in the area, we were familiar with the doctors at the various clinics and hospitals, so, when we found someone's problem required surgery or hospitalization, we would get on the phone and explain the situation to the physician or surgeon. With their agreement and that of their business offices, we were able to provide the patient care by someone who was able to admit patients, do surgery, and have their own liability insurance coverage. The actual cost-savings for evaluating and treating the patients referred to us who do not require hospital admission or surgery are truly significant. For example, it might cost a patient anywhere from $150 to $300 dollars to be seen by an orthopedic surgeon for a consultation, depending on the complexity of the evaluation. That fee plus the cost of lab and X-ray services, such as an MRI or CT scan, which the patient does not have to pay for, can add up to over one thousand dollars. Obviously, that would take a huge bite out of our patients' budgets if they had to come up with the money. More often than not, these patients choose not to see a doctor rather than incur such an expense, which results in the condition becoming much more difficult and costly to treat.

Initially, we saw patients one day a week, even though Kathy Williams was in the clinic three days a week to take phone calls and schedule patient appointments. Our clinic provides specialists in sixteen different medical and surgical fields. These include pediatrics, pediatric neurology, adult neurology, gastroenterology, internal medicine, allergy, endocrinology, nephrology, rheumatology, hematology, gynecology, orthopedic surgery, general surgery, podiatry, dermatology, and psychiatry.

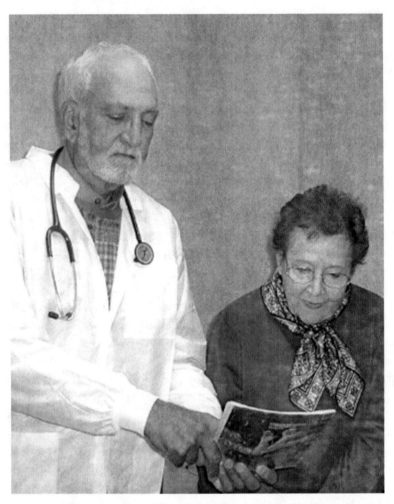

Figure 20 Teaching and consulting patients and medical students at BSP
Free Clinic

After a couple years of operation, we added ophthalmology and urology. We initially divided the specialties into groups of four so that each group would have clinic at least once a month. However, we found that the demands in internal medicine, psychiatry, and orthopedics made it necessary to schedule patients in those fields from monthly to at least twice a month. We soon grew out of the space initially allotted us on the third floor of a building the foundation had been leasing. We ended up converting a space in the basement of that building used to store records into our own space by moving the records elsewhere. This allowed us to have three examining rooms, a reception area, and a small conference room. Our patient numbers were initially disappointing, considering anywhere from 7 to 12 percent of the population in southcentral Wisconsin is uninsured. The problem was getting our clinic before the public and reminding doctors and clinics of the services we were able to provide.

After approximately a year of clinic operation, when we had seen about five hundred patients, the newspapers ran a human-interest story on the BSP Free Clinic. They came to the clinic, talked to patients, and took a number of photos which were used in the article. This publication was very important, as we did not have any kind of advertising budget, something I did not think we needed. On the other hand, before we could reach out to various sources of public and private revenue to serve our patients and meet our various budgetary needs, it was important to get some exposure in the media. We arranged to have Dr. Sundstrom and another volunteer appear on a TV spot and to talk about our project on a local radio talk show. Dr. George Roggensack, a retired radiologist, believed strongly in what we were doing. While we did not have our own X-ray department, he was willing to read our X-rays at the other hospitals if they would allow him to do so. More importantly, he agreed to head a fund-raising committee to approach sources of possible donations.

The initial responses he got from a number of the people were enthusiastically positive. He found out a few weeks later that enthusiasm had waned. It became apparent that something had happened that had caused this change in their interest. While we had no direct evidence, we surmised that those in the community who depended on health-care donations for their own operations saw us as competition and had contacted these people. We eventually came to realize that the door to United Way as a source of help had been closed, with no real explanation.

I decided that if several of us could talk to various groups in the community we might be able to garner some financial support from them. I was able to speak to physicians groups at both St. Mary's Hospital and Meriter Hospital and spoke at a South Madison Rotary Club luncheon. Dr. Sundstrom spoke at a downtown Rotary Club luncheon and a university physicians group. Many of the individual volunteer physicians contributed as much as one thousand dollars each to the fund drive, and, as it turns out, over half of the contributions to our project were raised from physicians in the community. This is due in part to a letter sent by the Dane County Medical Society to its members recommending the BSP Free Clinic for support. We got additional exposure when the *Wisconsin State Medical*

Journal published an editorial I wrote about physician-volunteer opportunities, which included my experience in Africa and getting the free clinic started.

Another area of frustration and controversy in fulfilling the BSP Free Clinic's mission in the first couple of years was that Jeanan Yasiri, who had been so helpful to me initially in getting the project from concept to reality, now appeared to be creating problems for our clinic coordinator, Kathy Williams. This was something I could never have imagined happening.

Among the various sources of patients coming to us from private doctor referrals was the Dean Clinic itself. A number of the family doctors and a few of the internists from the Dean Clinic had been referring their patients for consultations when they were aware of the financial stress some of their patients had. What was happening at the Dean Clinic was that the nurses of these referring doctors were being asked to make appointments to our clinic for their needy patients. Kathy, who would be on the phone with these nurses, eventually became familiar with them. In her enthusiasm for making it as easy as possible for them to refer to us, she typed up a memo describing what patients were and were not eligible to be seen and what services we had to offer. She also asked for any suggestions they might have to make them happier with the way things were being done.

This memo was sent to the nursing supervisors of the various Dean Clinic departments and eventually got into Jeanan Yasiri's hands. She apparently took offense and was upset enough to call Kathy to tell her never to do that again. She also said Dean Clinic doctors were not supposed to send us any patients because the clinic had its own community care program, but of course had the capacity to admit patients to the hospital and perform surgery. A large percentage of the doctors at the clinic did not think we were competing with Yasiri's pet project, and some were surprised at her reaction when told about it. Unfortunately, the president of the clinic, Dr. Allen Kemp, supported Jeanan, and that information came to us in the form of an impersonal memorandum.

The situation of a Dean Foundation–supported BSP Free Clinic being reprimanded by the Dean Medical Center created a level of tension that made many of us at the BSP Free Clinic uncomfortable. This was particularly true when it was rumored that the clinic had asked the foundation to gradually terminate its association with us and support for us. Fortunately, time has a way of healing wounds, and, while Kathy's zeal was dampened by the whole situation, she continued to drum up as much support as possible. Eventually, the same doctors began to refer patients to us because the medical reports they got from us were every bit as professional as those they got from other sources. In addition, the positive feedback they got from the patients they referred to us made them feel satisfied with our work. We subsequently agreed to reimburse the foundation for the salary and benefits Kathy was getting and to pay rent for the space we were using.

While accomplishing this has not been very easy, we have been getting better each year at attaining that goal, in large part due to the outstanding communication Kathy has had with anyone who has contributed time or money to our project. She has produced a quarterly newsletter full of pictures of various volunteers that keeps people up to date with how much we are accomplishing and makes this seem more of a family operation than some impersonal bureaucratic entity. I have had winter-holiday gatherings as well as a recent summer picnic at my home for all of the nonmedical and medical volunteers. Many brought salads and desserts with them. I guess in a way we have become a large family of volunteer health-care providers.

A major asset to maintaining the viability of the clinic has been the board of advisors established because of our business plan. The members consist of several physicians and dedicated prominent members of the university and business community. Their input has been particularly valuable in achieving our recent success in attaining some financial independence from the Dean Foundation. One example was the recommendation of putting on a talent show with community doctors providing the entertainment. This production not only sold out but also was very successful in helping us to raise funds.

Our service area covers southcentral Wisconsin, and at times patients coming to us do not have cars of their own and must depend on friends to get them to our facility. We have had about a 15 to 20 percent no-show rate (i.e., patients who are scheduled to see us not coming in for their appointments). We tried to reduce this figure by calling them the day of their appointment to remind them, but that has not changed the percentage a great deal. I have subsequently learned that this percentage is common, not only for free clinics but also for community health clinics in general. During the winter months, I have spent time in Florida, where I have obtained a license. The clinic in North Port, FL, where I volunteer has a similar no-show rate. The following brief story is an example of how we have tried to reduce the problem of no-shows at the BSP Free Clinic. One day we received a call from a patient who had an appointment to see us, and she told us the car a friend was using to take her to the appointment had broken down on the way to the clinic. Kathy Williams, who took the call, asked where the breakdown had occurred, and it was about two miles from the clinic. Kathy got in her car, picked up the patient, and brought her to the clinic. The driver was eventually able to get roadside help. As it worked out, the car was ready by the time she had seen me at the clinic for her orthopedic problem and was ready to go home.

Our clinic continues to attract volunteer physicians who retire every year and who would like to participate in our mission. It is my hope that someday our health-care system will provide medical care for every person, regardless of whether they are employed. I am not certain that a Canadian system would work here, given the fact that so many Canadians come to this country for care because of significant flaws in their system. This system involves quotas for a number of particular surgeries and has limits on expensive diagnostic procedures and treatments. Their recent acknowledgment that the delays caused by such practices have resulted in the unnecessary deaths of some Canadians is unacceptable. Now their judicial courts have finally recognized the problem and are allowing Canadians to buy their own private health insurance if they so desire. This was something that was not possible until recently. I am not sure we need to eliminate the private health insurance sector in America and replace it with a government system, but I do think a government system or a private system, similar to Kaiser Permanente, supported with federal funds will be needed to achieve universal medical health coverage. This would likely result in a "Cadillac and Volkswagen" form of health care. Either option eventually gets us to the destination, which is better than our current system. Having volunteer citizens serve on boards that would oversee complaints that might arise from either program would be an important element to make certain individuals are not buried in the bureaucracies of any government program when it comes to drug and treatment benefits.

Postscript

It has not been my intention to shock or scare readers by initially dwelling on a few bad or unethical doctors. Fortunately, I believe there are not great numbers as flagrant as the few examples I used. While huge egos and idiosyncrasies make some individuals stand out more than others, they do not harm patients if they practice ethical medicine. This does not mean they are not difficult to work with at times, but that is usually a small price to pay for quality medicine. As Hippocrates advised centuries ago, a major tenet of ethical medicine is to do no harm to our patients, particularly because of greed or incompetence.

A major part of the education of medical students, interns, and residents, regardless of their medical specialty, should be to teach compassion and understanding of the needs and concerns of patients. It is critical that the medical care we provide not only meets the physical but also the psychological needs of the patient. Doctors become particularly aware of this when they become patients themselves. I constantly look to see if caregivers are making eye contact with me or just focused on their computer, now that we have electronic records. We must not let technology make us insensitive to the kind of personal relationships doctors and their patients had for decades.

If aspiring doctors and educators come away with some concepts from reading the observations I have made, I will have accomplished half of my goal. At the same time, if the public understands some of the ways they can evaluate their physicians, realizing they are not perfect, then the remaining half of my goal will have been accomplished as well. Thank you for allowing me to take you on my personal journey to become a physician and practice the specialty of orthopedic surgery. I hope your knowledge and understanding have been enriched by reading it.

Glossary of Medical Terms and Phrases

1. Amnesia: loss of memory

2. Aneurysm: abnormal bulging or enlargement of a blood vessel

3. Apgar Score: measurement of a newborn response to birth

4. Arterio-venous fistula: abnormal connection between an artery and vein bypassing the flow of blood through capillaries

5. Articulation: the junction between two or more bones

6. Arthroplasty: surgical restoration of a joint with natural or artificial materials

7. Arthroscope: a cylindrical instrument used to visualize the inside of a joint

8. Arthroscopic debridement: removal of bone chips, spurs, and frayed cartilage from a joint using an arthroscope to see the inside of the joint

9. Biomechanics: the application of mechanical laws to living structures

10. Biopsy: removal of a small piece of tissue or bone to be examined under a microscope to make a diagnosis

11. Bone cortex: outer layer of a bone

12. Bunion: bony prominence at the level of the first joint of the big toe

13. Bunionectomy: operation to remove a bunion

14. Bronchus: either of the two main branches of the trachea (windpipe)

15. Bronchi: plural of bronchus

16. Calcaneus: the heel bone, one of the tarsal bones of the foot

17. Capillaries: smallest vessels to transport blood

18. Causalgia: burning pain due to a wound or other injury to a peripheral nerve

19. Collateral ligaments: ligaments located on the left and right sides of a joint

20. Consults: patients a specialist is asked to evaluate and/or treat

21. Contractures: shortening or shrinkage of ligaments and muscles around a joint

22. Craniotomy: removal of a portion of the skull to expose the brain

23. Cuboid: cube-shaped bone in the middle of the foot, a tarsal bone

24. Curet: a kind of scraper or spoon for removing growths or tissue from walls of cavities

25. Curettage: the use of, or treatment by, the curet

26. Disarticulation: amputation or separation at a joint

27. Dissecting: cutting, separating, and exposing body parts

28. Distal: lower end of a bone

29. Exsanguinate: to deprive of blood

30. External fixator: a device made up of a combination of pins placed into bone through skin and connected to rods to stabilize broken bones

31. Fasciotomy: cutting the fascia, which is fibrous tissue surrounding groups and individual muscle

32. Femur: thigh bone

33. Fibula: smaller of the two bones in the leg

34. Fistula: abnormal passage leading to a hollow organ or cavity

35. Flexor hallucis longus tendon: the structure that bends the big toe

36. GP: general practitioner; family doctor

37. Gram Stain: a method developed by a Danish physician Hans Christian Gram to identify bacteria

38. Hospitalist: specialist who accepts the responsibility for other doctors' patients who are admitted to the hospital

39. Hysterectomy: surgery to remove the uterus

40. Hysterical paralysis: apparent but not real paralysis brought on by emotional problems

41. Lamina of the spine: flattened area of the vertebra that forms the roof of the spinal canal

42. Lateral meniscus: cartilage pad on the outer side of the knee

43. Lumbar: the lower back between the last rib and the pelvis

44. Lumbar laminectomy: removal of part or all of the lamina of lumbar vertebra

45. Meconium: bile-stained contents of the fetal intestine

46. Mitosis: cells dividing

47. Necrosis: death of tissue and/or organs

48. Osteomyelitis: bone infection

49. Osteotome: a chisel used to cut bone

50. Osteotomy: surgically cutting through bone, often used to correct a deformity

51. Palpate: to touch or feel with one's hands

52. Permanent residuals: physical changes resulting from trauma or disease that are not likely to change

53. Plate fixation: use of a metal plate and screws to hold a broken bone together

54. Pneumo-encephalogram: type of X-ray done to show the fluid-filled areas of the brain by replacing the fluid with air

55. Popliteal artery: a major artery located behind the knee

56. Postdatism: the period of time after the expected due date for a pregnancy

57. Proximal: the upper end of a bone

58. Proximal tibial osteotomy: bone cut made completely through the tibia just below the knee

59. Pseudoparalysis: apparent but not a real paralysis

60. Psychosomatic: having bodily symptoms of an emotional or mental origin

61. Pubic symphysis: the articulation of the left and right pubic bones made up fibrous and cartilage tissue

62. Sacrum: fusion of five vertebra located between the left and right half of the back of the pelvis

63. Septicemia: serious and potentially lethal condition resulting from the presence of bacteria and their associated toxins in the blood

64. Tarsal: related to the bones of the arch of the foot

65. Vasopressor: drug used to raise blood pressure

66. Workup: the evaluation of a patient by taking a history, doing a physical examination, and ordering appropriate tests

978-0-595-47934-₄
0-595-47934-0

Printed in the United States
115863LV00001B/209/P